OXFORD MEDICAL PUBLICATIONS

World blindness and its prevention

Volume 2

World blindness and its prevention

Volume 2

Edited by
the International Agency for the Prevention of Blindness
under the direction of Sir John Wilson

The IAPB wishes to acknowledge the contribution made by
Ann Darnbrough to the compilation and editing of this book

Oxford New York Toronto
OXFORD UNIVERSITY PRESS
1984

Oxford University Press, Walton Street, Oxford OX2 6DP

London Glasgow New York Toronto
Delhi Bombay Calcutta Madras Karachi
Kuala Lumpur Singapore Hong Kong Tokyo
Nairobi Dar es Salaam Cape Town
Melbourne Auckland

and associates in
Beirut Berlin Ibdan Mexico City Nicosia

Oxford is a trade mark of Oxford University Press

© *The International Agency for*
the Prevention of Blindness, 1984

All rights reserved. No part of this publication may be reproduced, stored in a retrieval system, or transmitted, in any form or by any means, electronic, mechanical, photocopying, recording, or otherwise, without the prior permission of Oxford University Press

British Library Cataloguing in Publication Data

World blindness and its prevention.
  Vol. 2
  1. Blindness—Prevention
  I. Wilson, Sir John, 1919-   II. International
  Agency for the Prevention of Blindness
  617.7'12   RE91
  ISBN 0-19-261480-0

Library of Congress Cataloging in Publication Data

(Revised for volume 2)
Main entry under title:
World blindness and its prevention.
  (Oxford medical publications)
  Includes index.
  1. Blindness—Prevention.   I. Wilson, John, Sir,
1919-   II. International Agency for the Prevention
of Blindness. [DNLM: 1. Blindness—Congresses.
2. Blindness—Prevention and control—Congresses.
3. International cooperation—Congresses.   WW 276 W927
1982]
RE91.W67   617.7'12052   79-41190
ISBN 0-19-261480-0

Set by Joshua Asociates, Oxford
Printed in Great Britain by the Thetford Press, Norfolk

At least half of all blindness in the world is preventable. The IAPB, with its national and international partners, seeks to reduce the global toll of 40 million blind people by increasing awareness of this problem among the people of the world and their governments, by encouraging financial and manpower support of blindness prevention programmes, and by promoting the development of effective prevention programmes employing the most appropriate and economic technology.

Preface

This book brings together some of the papers presented at the Second General Assembly of the International Agency for the Prevention of Blindness (IAPB) held in Bethesda, Maryland, USA from 25 to 28 October 1982. These have, however, been increased in scope and significance by expanding and updating the documents and by the inclusion of further relevant material.

The book seeks not only to review what is happening throughout the world to prevent blindness, but considers the measures necessary to join effectively with the World Health Organization in meeting the goal of 'Health for All by the Year 2000'. Dr Carl Kupfer, the new President of IAPB, emphasizes that the Agency must address itself to future problems in world blindness as well as present realities. 'For the future incidence and distribution of blinding eye diseases will determine what resources we must expend in order to reduce the global toll of blindness over the next two decades and thereafter.'

Eye diseases which will assume greater importance in the future include cataract, glaucoma, and other disorders associated with ageing. Because life expectancy is rising in both the developed and the developing countries, the incidence of these ageing-related eye disorders is also increasing. The consequences of this trend are enormous. For example, in the United States the prevalence of cataract, glaucoma, and senile macular degeneration among people 55 and older is expected to increase by more than 150 per cent between now and the year 2030. In the developing countries, a similar surge in ageing-related eye disease can be predicted from demographic trends: the number of people aged 55 and over is expected to increase fivefold in these countries by the year 2025.

Thus we can anticipate a massive, world-wide increase in several blinding diseases unless new methods of prevention are found. While the world's vision researchers seek the needed preventive measures, the IAPB and its national blindness prevention committees must attempt to ensure that health care systems are prepared to deal with the projected upsurge in ageing-related eye disease if it occurs. Through planning and determination, we can reduce world blindness in spite of the dangerous trends that threaten to increase it.

Contents

List of contributors	xi
1 A global perspective *R. Muller*	1
2 Six main causes of blindness *C. Kupfer*	4
Trachoma	4
Xerophthalmia	5
Onchocerciasis	7
Cataract	8
Glaucoma	10
Ocular trauma	12
3 Retrospect *Sir John Wilson*	14
4 Regional action	18
Africa	18
Eastern Europe	24
Latin America	29
The Middle East	32
North America	36
South-East Asia	40
Southern Asia	43
Western Europe	49
Western Pacific	50
5 Development of national programmes	55
How to develop a national programme *Madan Mohan*	55
Eye health care delivery systems *Robert H. Meaders*	60
Personnel training *M. C. Chirambo*	67
Kenya Rural Blindness Prevention Project *R. Whitfield, Jr*	69
Evaluation of blindness prevention programmes *F. Hollows*	74
Programme for the prevention and control of blindness in Nepal *R. Pararajasegaram*	78
Primary eye-care programme in the eastern region of Peru *Francisco Contreras*	82
Practical problems and successes of the RCSB cataract surgery programme in India *Rajendra Vyas*	85
The control of xerophthalmia in Indonesia *I. Tarwotjo and R. Tilden*	86
Training and role of primary eye-care technicians in Guatemala *Gloria Tujab*	89
Survey and treatment of the blind in Zhong-Shan County, Guang-Dong, China *Mao Wen-shu, Chen Yao-Zhen, and Guan Sheng-shi*	92
6 Resource mobilization	95
Economic justification and implications for the prevention of blindness *J. H. Costello*	95
Availability of and need for development of multinational resources within a region *R. Pararajasegaram*	97
Mobilization of bilateral resources *A. T. Jenkyns*	102
The role of philanthropy in resource mobilization *K. L. Stumpf*	103
Fund raising *W. Stein*	107

The development of governmental and inter-governmental
   resources *Dorina de Gouvea Nowill*   108
Communications, publicity, and public relations *Jean Wilson*   110

Epilogue *Carl Kupfer*   114

Supplements   116

A. WHO Collaborating Centres for the Prevention of Blindness   116
B. International non-governmental organizations   117
Brief reports presented by: The Asian Foundation, Christoffel Blindenmission, Foresight, Helen Keller International, International Eye Foundation, International Glaucoma Association, Operation Eyesight Universal, Royal Commonwealth Society for the Blind, Seva Foundation.

Appendix

I Officers of the Agency, Members of the Executive Board, and Chairmen of regional Committees   129

Appendix

II Participation at the Second General Assembly in Washington DC, USA   133

Index   135

Contributors

Sheik Abdullah M. Al-Ghanim, Chairman, The Regional Bureau of the Middle East Committee for the Welfare of the Blind, Riyadh, Saudi Arabia.
Dr F. Billson, Department of Clinical Ophthalmology, Sydney Eye Hospital, Woolloomooloo, Australia.
Mrs Virginia Boyce, National Society to Prevent Blindness, New York, USA.
Professor Chen Yao-Shen, The Eye Hospital of Zhong-Shan Medical College, Guangzhou, Guang-Dong Province, China.
Dr M. C. Chirambo, Chief Medical Officer, Ministry of Health, Lilongwe, Malawi.
Dr Viggo Clemmesen, Central Hospital, Naestved, Denmark.
Dr Francisco Contreras, Director, Centro Oftalmologico, Hospital Santo Toribio de Mogrovejo, Lima, Peru.
J. H. Costello, Director, Helen Keller International, New York, USA.
Dr C. Dawson, Director, Francis I. Proctor Foundation for Research in Ophthalmology, University of California, San Francisco, California, USA.
Dorina de Gouvea Nowill, President, World Council for the Welfare of the Blind, Sao Paulo, Brazil.
Professor F. Hollows, Department of Ophthalmology, Prince of Wales Hospital, Randwick, New South Wales, Australia.
A. T. Jenkyns, President, Operation Eyesight Universal, Calgary, Alberta, Canada.
Dr Carl Kupfer, President, International Agency for the Prevention of Blindness, National Eye Institute, Bethesda, Maryland, USA.
Dr A. Lim, Mount Elizabeth Medical Centre, Singapore.
Dr Erik Linner, Head, Department of Ophthalmology, University of Gothenburg, Sahlgran's Hospital, Gothenburg, Sweden.
Dr Robert H. Meaders, Medical Director, International Eye Foundation, Bethesda, Maryland, USA.
Professor Madan Mohan, Professor of Ophthalmology and Chief Organizer of the Dr Rajendra Prasad Centre for Ophthalmic Sciences, All India Institute of Medical Sciences, New Delhi, India.
Robert Muller, Assistant Secretary General, United Nations, New York, USA.
Dr R. Pararajasegaram, Medical Officer Prevention of Blindness, South-East Asian Regional Office, World Health Organization, New Delhi, India.
Professor C. O. Quarcoopome, Medical Officer Prevention of Blindness—Africa Region, c/o World Health Co-ordinator, Lilongwe, Malawi.
Associate Professor Guan Sheng-Shi, The Eye Hospital of Zhong-Shan Medical College, Guangzhou, Guang-Dong Province, China.
Dr A. Sommer, Director, International Centre for Epidemiologic and Preventive Ophthalmology, The Wilmer Institute, Baltimore, Maryland, USA.
W. Stein, Head of Overseas Division, Christoffel-Blindenmission, Bensheim, Federal Republic of Germany.
Dr K. L. Stumpf, Executive Director, Asian Foundation for the Prevention of Blindness, Kowloon, Hong Kong.
Dr I. Tarwotjo, Director Nutrition Unit, Ministry of Health, Jakarta, Indonesia.
Dr R. Tilden, Programme Officer, Helen Keller International, New York, USA.
Gloria Tujab, Primary Eye Care Technician, National Committee for the Blind and the Deaf of Guatemala, Guatemala City, Guatemala.
Dr Rajendra T. Vyas, Asia Director, Royal Commonwealth Society for the Blind, Bombay, India.
Professor Mao Wen-Shu, The Eye Hospital of Zhong-Shan Medical College, Guangzhou, Guang-Dong Province, China.

Dr R. Whitfield, Jr., Director, Kenya Rural Blindness Prevention Project, Nyeri, Kenya.

Lady Jean Wilson, Deputy Director (UK Activities), Royal Commonwealth Society for the Blind, Haywards Heath, UK.

Sir John Wilson, Honorary President, International Agency for the Prevention of Blindness, Haywards Heath, UK.

Colonel Boris Zimin, President of the World Council for the Welfare of the Blind, Moscow, USSR.

1

A global perspective
R. Muller

On the occasion of the Second General Assembly of the International Agency for the Prevention of Blindness, Dr Robert Muller, Assistant Secretary-General of the United Nations, delivered the keynote address. We are privileged to reproduce the main points of his speech in which he provided a historical and global perspective to the subject of prevention of disability in general and prevention of blindness in particular.

I am very honoured indeed to be bringing to you the personal greetings of the Secretary-General of the United Nations, Mr Perez de Cuellar and of Mr Bradford Morse, the Director of the United Nations Development Programme. It is significant that this meeting is taking place during the precise week when the United Nations General Assembly will be adopting the programme of action for the handicapped. A programme arising as a direct result of the International Year of Disabled Persons.

My function in the United Nations involves an awareness of new problems, as well as co-ordination, and having a dynamic sense of what the 32 world programmes and specialized agencies are doing. I am thus in a good position to recognize the benefits that the UN as a universal organization can bring to the many and interrelated problems of this planet.

To put the subject of health strategies into historical perspective we need to remember that until 1951 we did not even have an accurate figure for the world population. It took until the early 1970s for all the data on the world population to be collected at a time when the population had increased from $2\frac{1}{2}$ billion to almost 4 billion people. The world promptly awoke to the fact that a host of global problems was emerging everywhere, that there were vast numbers of people in certain categories who needed help. Suddenly there was a world environment crisis, a food crisis, then an energy crisis; one after another the massive problems had to be confronted. Until that time nobody had any idea of the vast scale of the problems.

It was about 1970 that we discovered through UNESCO that there were 350 million handicapped people on this planet. It was then that the United Nations became aware of the need to prevent disability. Until that time, the help that had been made available was no more than an attempt to meet the immediate perceived need, and largely in the field of rehabilitation—helping people to make wheelchairs and crutches.

The new problems discovered at this time were of frightening magnitude. At a time when in the industrialized countries we had been able to eradicate most of the communicable diseases, the population explosion in the developing countries, where such diseases had yet to be conquered, was leading to a phenomenal increase in handicap. At the same time, in the industrialized countries, a different cause of handicap was emerging as the major source of disability, with as many as 50 million accidents occurring each year in factories and another 7½ million on the roads—250 000 of them fatal. Inevitably, it was realized that this devastating trend would in time spread to developing countries. We were, in fact, moving on two fronts towards a world disaster of the worst magnitude. In response to this realization, it became essential both to warn people of the problems and also to take action to avert a catastrophe. This was, in fact, the impetus for the International Year of Disabled Persons in 1981.

In the meantime, however, the number of handicapped people was steadily rising, and there was need for positive intervention to minimize the disaster. I was, therefore, in 1975, happy to find on my desk a press release from the World Health Organization announcing the creation of IAPB. I was happy because it meant that for one component of the world's handicapped, namely the blind, the world community was organizing itself in order to launch a global campaign for the prevention of one of the world's major handicaps. A handicap which is estimated to affect between 26 million and 42 million people according to the definition which is taken of either total blindness or seriously impaired vision. The Agency was created as an international initiative and as part of the effort to grasp a growing global problem.

It is integrated within the plan of the World Health Organization to achieve certain objectives by the year 2000, alongside other plans—world literacy, world population, world employment, world environment.

IAPB is also a component of the draft plan of action for the handicapped, adopted by the United Nations. It is a beautiful plan. I think it is the first time in the history of the world that the human species has set down its targets and goals for 450 million of its brothers and sisters. Within this general plan we need to have a sub-strategy for the prevention and cure of blindness. This strategy must take into account a growing problem—the ageing of the world population. As ageing increases throughout the world, the number of blind people will also increase. The problem will be much greater for the developing countries in 30 or 40 years from now than it is in the West, because the longevity of their huge populations is rapidly improving. The consequential problems may indeed be such that by the year 2000 there may be even more blind people in the world than there are today.

It is, therefore, essential to develop a systematic world strategy with an intensification of research and technology in the developing countries. I am happy to learn that the World Health Organization has created a Programme Advisory Group on the prevention of blindness, and is involved with setting up 11 Collaborating Centres for the prevention of blindness, in order to have a co-ordinated system of research on specific diseases and prevention. Scientific and technological research is, at present, too heavily concentrated in the north, and resources need to be transferred to developing countries.

I regard prevention as the most important activity the international community can undertake. Given the size of the problem, large-scale prevention of disability is the most promising avenue of approach. I can tell you that if I were ever offered a post as Minister of Health, I would refuse unless the title included 'prevention'—Minister of Health and Prevention.

Prevention of blindness programmes, to be successful, need the co-operation of non-governmental organizations who are prepared to work together, and with governments. I believe IAPB can be a model for what can be done in many other fields. I can tell you that you will receive every possible help from the United Nations system.

In conclusion let me talk about vision in a broader perspective. When I take the field of vision, the scope of our eyesight, I would almost like to propose that the World Health Organization and UNESCO should try to come up with a total figure of world expenditure on vision. The human species has been able to extend its vision a million times over. We have been able to enlarge the infinitely small with microscopes, electronic microscopes, and now picoscopes. We have immense cyclotrons so that we can see the subparticles and particles of matter. And we have been able to extend our vision into the infinite, into the outer reaches of space with ever more sophisticated telescopes. I think it would be of interest to the international community to know what these efforts cost. We might find the figures staggering: that we spend much more in order to see particles and subparticles, and to look at far-away planets and galaxies, then we spend on the few millions of our brothers and sisters who do not even have normal scope of vision. Such an investigation could well lessen the distortion of our priorities.

We have developed our physical capacities, our sensorial capacities, and our mental capacities, but now we are confronted in the United Nations with an even more fundamental fact—that we have not even begun to develop our sentimental faculties—the faculties of the heart, the faculties of helping each other, the faculties of loving each other, the faculty of respecting the dignity of each human being. Our capacity for seeing can benefit enormously if we can also develop our capacities for understanding and for mutual co-operation.

2

Six main causes of blindness
C. Kupfer

This chapter contains statements about the six main causes of blindness. Each statement is followed by a distillate of the general recommendations agreed at the IAPB Second General Assembly, for national committees to use in promoting appropriate prevention of blindness programmes in their own countries.

TRACHOMA

Definition

Trachoma is a highly contagious bacterial disease that affects about 500 million people world-wide. Approximately 6 to 9 million are blind from trachoma and another 100 million have serious visual impairment that may progress to blindness. The disease is most common in the drier regions of the developing countries. It is particularly frequent in Africa, the Middle East, the Indian subcontinent, and parts of South-East Asia.

Trachoma is associated with poverty, overcrowding, lack of clean water, and poor sanitation. Under suitable conditions, the disease spreads rapidly.

Early signs of trachoma include reddening, burning, and watering of the eyes. These signs are caused by irritation of the conjunctiva, and may subside. However, if the infection is left untreated, it gradually causes inflammation of the cornea. The most serious corneal damage occurs when the eyelids become inverted, so that the eyelashes rub against the cornea. This abrasion can cause corneal ulcers, perforations, and scarring, which may result in blindness.

Although infection with the trachoma-causing bacterium (*Chlamydia trachomatis*) usually occurs in childhood, visual loss most often happens during adult years. In many cases, blindness does not result until 10 to 20 years after the initial infection.

Trachoma can be treated effectively with topically administered antibiotics and other drugs. However, unless the environmental factors that favour the spread of the disease are corrected, the infection may recur.

Progress

Trachoma has been eliminated already from the most developed regions of the world through the improvement in living conditions that has accompanied industrialization. In other areas where trachoma remains endemic, community-wide control programmes based on the mass application of topical antibiotics, accompanied by environmental health measures, have been found effective in reducing the frequency and severity of the disease. None the less, the continuing toll of visual loss from trachoma indicates a need for more extensive efforts to combat this disease.

Strategy

Participants in the workshop on trachoma at the Assembly of the IAPB suggested the following strategy for control of the disease:

1. Systematic assessment programmes should be used to identify communities where blinding trachoma is endemic.
2. High priority should be assigned to detecting trachoma and reducing its prevalence amongst young children.
3. Mass treatment with topical tetracycline should be undertaken in any community where the prevalence of trachoma amongst children is 20 per cent or more.
4. Adults should be included along with children in trachoma screening programmes.
5. Screening should be designed to identify cases of trichiasis and entropion (the sight-threatening eyelid deformities caused by trachoma) requiring surgery. The effectiveness of this surgery should be assessed.
6. Attention should be given to non-medical measures that can reduce the incidence of trachoma. These include economic development and improvement of water supplies and sanitation.

XEROPHTHALMIA (BLINDING MALNUTRITION)

Definition

Xerophthalmia is a potentially blinding eye disease associated with vitamin-A deficiency. The disorder is prevalent among malnourished children in developing countries and is a leading cause of childhood blindness world-wide. In Asia alone, it is estimated that about 5 million children each year develop early signs of xerophthalmia, and in 250 000 of these children, the disease may become severe enough to cause blindness.

In xerophthalmia, vitamin-A deficiency causes dryness of the exposed surface of the eye. This early form of xerophthalmia can be reversed by providing the affected child with adequate amounts of vitamin A or its precursors. If these measures are not taken, the child is at risk of developing a more severe form of xerophthalmia in which a rapid softening of the cornea occurs. Within hours of the onset of this condition, called keratomalacia, corneal ulceration and perforation may occur, resulting in loss of vision and perhaps in destruction of the eye. Keratomalacia is most likely to occur in those vitamin-A-deficient children who also suffer from severe protein deficiency or an infectious disease such as measles.

Progress

Xerophthalmia has disappeared from the industrialized countries, largely because of nutritional improvements brought about by the overall rise in the standard of living. Also, many of the developing nations, such as some in East Africa, have few cases of the disease because the diet traditionally consumed by children and nursing mothers contains dark green leafy vegetables or other foods rich in precursors of vitamin A. In the remaining countries, where xerophthalmia is a major public health problem, efforts to prevent blindness from the disease have centred on raising the level of vitamin A in the entire population, or in nutritionally deprived groups. For example, Guatemala has succeeded in increasing the vitamin-A intake of its people through a programme involving fortification of a basic foodstuff, sugar. In other countries—such as Indonesia, India, and Bangladesh—vitamin-A concentrate has been delivered to susceptible infants and children in liquid or capsule form. Although these mass distribution programmes have been highly successful in preventing or reversing vitamin-A deficiency in the children treated, their effectiveness has been blunted by difficulties in reaching the children at greatest risk of blindness. Recently there has been considerable progress in improving the design of such programmes, with emphasis being placed on identifying—or targeting—the segment of the population at greatest risk for xerophthalmia. Also, nutrition education programmes for mothers of children at risk, and training programmes for health car workers, are being integrated into the overall prevention effort wherever possible.

Strategy

Participants in the xerophthalmia workshop at the Assembly made the following recommendations:

1. More must be learned about measles blindness and its relationship to xerophthalmia, particular in Africa.
2. Oral vitamin-A concentrate must be made available to all countries where xerophthalmia is prevalent.
3. All health workers in these countries must be trained to recognize and treat xerophthalmia.
4. Studies must be carried out to determine why high-risk children are not consuming leafy green vegetables and other vitamin-A-rich food.
5. The effort to identify and initiate appropriate interventions against xerophthalmia must continue. Examples of such interventions include:
    (a) distribution of vitamin A to all children with high-risk or predisposing factors for xerophthalmia;

(b) integration of screening and treatment for xerophthalmia with appropriate health education as part of the service provided by eye camps; and

(c) instruction of village midwives in the administration of tetracycline and vitamin A. In high-risk communities, 50 000 IU of vitamin A should be administered orally to each infant and 200 000 IU to the mother at the time of the infant's birth or shortly thereafter.

ONCHOCERCIASIS

Definition

Onchocerciasis, also known as 'river blindness', is a parasitic disease that affects an estimated 20 to 30 million people. About 1 million are blind from the disorder. The prevalence of onchocerciasis is highest in tropical Africa, where up to 50 per cent of the inhabitants in some villages can be affected. The disease is also found in Yemen and in Central and South America.

The parasite responsible for onchocerciasis is *Onchocerca volvulus*, a worm of the filaria group. It is transmitted from person to person by the bite of a river-breeding insect, the black-fly *Simulium*. When a person is bitten by a fly carrying *Onchocerca*, the worms concentrate in nodules in or under the skin and eventually produce millions of embryos called microfilariae. These migrate throughout the tissues of the victim, showing a preference for the skin and the eyes. Ocular lesions caused by the microfilariae may result in blindness. Usually this eye damage progresses slowly, and severe visual impairment may not occur until a decade after the initial infection.

Treatment with drugs that kill *Onchocerca* worms or microfilariae often can halt the progression of onchocerciasis and prevent severe damage to the eye. Unfortunately, the preparations now available for this purpose have adverse side-effects and other limitations that render them unsuitable for use in mass treatment programmes.

Progress

Although large-scale control of onchocerciasis cannot presently be achieved by medical means, programmes designed to combat the disease by destroying the black-fly vector have been strikingly successful. Onchocerciasis was eliminated from Kenya as a result of a 1947 project which used DDT to kill *Simulium* larvae in the rivers. Recently, the Onchocerciasis Control Programme of the Volta River Basin Area has sharply reduced the incidence of onchocerciasis in an even larger region through an intensive effort to eradicate the black-fly. Aerial spraying of rivers with larvicides has resulted in control of *Simulium* in 80 per cent of the 3/4 million square kilometres covered by the programme. In most localities, virtually all children born since the programme began in 1975 are free of onchocerciasis. Prevention of new cases has brought about a marked decline in the prevalence of the disease as well, with a reduction of 20 per cent being noted in some areas.

Strategy

Participants in the onchocerciasis workshop at the Assembly made the following recommendations:

1. Much additional research must be conducted on onchocerciasis:
    (a) to determine the incidence of ocular lesions in this disease, discover how these lesions progress, and determine what factors favour their development;
    (b) to determine the routes by which the eye is invaded, using animal models;
    (c) to characterize the effects of the disease on ocular tissues;
    (d) to detect early retinal changes caused by the disease; flourescein angiography might be employed in these studies;
    (e) to develop a test for dark adaptation that can be used in the field; and
    (f) to develop a means of measuring visual fields that can be used outside a clinical setting.
2. Additional drugs must be developed for the treatment of onchocerciasis; in particular, there is a need for a new, safe drug to kill the adult worm.
3. Controlled trials should be carried out to determine the safety and efficacy of drugs currently available.
4. Techniques for diagnosis of onchocerciasis must be improved; in particular, immunodiagnostic methods must be developed to supplement existing diagnostic techniques.
5. New larvicides must be developed for the control of the black-fly.
6. All possible effort should be made to publicize the great achievement of the Onchocerciasis Control Programme in the Volta River Basin Area.

CATARACT

Definition

Cataract, an opacity or cloudiness in the normally clear lens of the eye that interferes with vision, is a major cause of blindness in the industrialized as well as the developing countries. World-wide, about 17 million people are blind from cataract. Millions of additional cases of the disorder occur each year, and in many countries its incidence appears to be rising.

The most common form of cataract is associated with ageing; this form is becoming more frequent as the average age of the world's population rises because of improvements in nutrition and health care. Other forms of cateract are caused by infection, inflammation, injury, genetic traits, and diabetes and other metabolic influences.

At present, cataract formation cannot be prevented. But blindness resulting from cataract can be reversed through surgery—one of the most successful of all major operations.

Problems and progress

Although cataract surgery is highly effective, its sight-saving potential has not been fully realized: world-wide, only about 10 to 20 per cent of all cataracts are removed. A shortage of trained medical personnel and facilities is the chief factor limiting the use of cataract surgery in developing nations. Another obstacle, common in the industrialized countries as well, is the reluctance of many cataract victims to undergo surgery.

Major efforts are being made to overcome the problems that limit utilization of cataract surgery in the developing countries. Through the use of mobile surgical units and/or temporary eye camps in several of these countries, the benefits of cataract surgery have been extended to large numbers of rural people who would otherwise have gone untreated. For example, in 1981 the Royal Commonwealth Society for the Blind sponsored 2300 eye camps on the Indian subcontinent. More than a million people were examined and treated in these camps, and almost 200 000 cataract operations were performed. Streamlining of preoperative and surgical procedures, along with introduction of recently developed surgical techniques such as cryoextraction, have increased the success rate of cataract surgeries performed in eye camps to as high as 90 to 95 per cent.

None the less, even in the countries where mobile units and eye camps have been used most extensively, these systems have not been sufficient to meet the need for cataract surgery among rural populations. Unless preventive measures for cataract are discovered and applied, health care planners in many countries will be confronted with the problem of how to expand the availability of cataract treatment fast enough to keep pace with the growing number of cases.

It is clear that some means of preventing or delaying the onset of cataract will be needed to reduce the prevalence of the disease. Such a breakthrough would be a major step in reducing world blindness.

Strategy

Participants in the cataract workshop at the Assembly made the following recommendations:

1. Suitable ophthalmic services must be established to keep pace with the increase in the number of people requiring cataract surgery and

to abolish the backlog of unoperated cases, particularly in Asia and Africa; epidemiological data should be used in planning the ophthalmic services.
2. Mobile eye units should be considered as a means of delivering these ophthalmic services when other facilities are inadequate; however, these mobile units should not be considered as a permanent solution to the problem of providing treatment for cataract.
3. International co-operation will be necessary to provide the resources for adequate ophthalmic services until each nation has achieved self-sufficiency in caring for its cataract victims.
4. Cataract surgery may be delegated to technically skilled non-physicians in exceptional circumstances; however, these technicians should be well trained and well supervised by an ophthalmologist, and their use should not be considered a permanent solution to the problem of providing adequate numbers of cataract surgeons.
5. New technology for the extraction of cataracts should be carefully evaluated.
6. Research on the mechanisms of cataract must be intensified so that methods of prevention and non-surgical treatment can be developed.
7. The IAPB should discourage marketing of alleged anti-cataract drugs until evidence of their effectiveness has been obtained.

GLAUCOMA

Definition

Glaucoma is visual loss associated with increased pressure within the eye. Although glaucoma can be treated and serious visual loss prevented in most cases, the disease is none the less a major cause of world blindness. Available estimates indicate that glaucoma is responsible for 11 per cent of all blindness in the United States, 20 per cent in Ghana and the People's Republic of China, and more than 30 per cent in Brazil. The most common form of the disease, chronic or open-angle glaucoma, is believed to be present in about 1 per cent of all people over the age of 40. (However, in some parts of South-East Asia, acute or angle-closure glaucoma is much more common.)

Chronic open-angle glaucoma develops gradually and painlessly, and is often unnoticed until a substantial amount of visual function is already lost. Fortunately, the elevated pressure can usually be controlled with periodic doses of medication, most often in the form of eyedrops, and blindness thereby prevented. For those cases which cannot be treated with drugs, surgery is often beneficial.

Progress and problems

Mass screening has played an important role in identifying unsuspecting glaucoma victims throughout the world. However, early detection remains one of the primary problems in preventing visual loss from this disease. In some countries there are two few doctors to provide adequate glaucoma screening and treatment programmes. Also, in many nations medical facilities are not easily accessible to people in remote areas.

Even among those identified as glaucoma patients, treatment poses a problem in some parts of the world because of difficulties in obtaining and storing anti-glaucoma drugs. In addition, many patients are unable or unwilling to use the eyedrops prescribed for the glaucoma, and some patients refuse needed surgery because they fear it. Laser treatment shows great promise as an alternative to conventional surgery, especially for angle-closure glaucoma, but the ophthalmic lasers now available are not suitable for use by field-workers in undeveloped rural areas.

Strategy

Participants in the glaucoma workshop at the Assembly made the following recommendations:

1. The distinction between open-angle and angle-closure glaucoma should be retained as a useful concept in designing glaucoma programmes.
2. Efforts must be made to detect angle-closure glaucoma as early as possible; health education programmes which teach people to recognize the symptoms of the disease can be helpful in bringing cases to medical attention.
3. If angle-closure glaucoma is detected early enough to save the vision in the first affected eye, that should be the initial goal of treatment. If most of the vision in this eye has been lost, however, the goal of treatment should be to provide prophylaxis for the second eye.
4. Open-angle glaucoma should be detected by examinations which combine determination of intraocular pressure and measurement of the visual field.
5. New instruments must be developed to facilitate the detection of open-angle glaucoma by primary health workers in the field. For example, a simple static perimeter that could be used under field conditions would be extremely valuable; simpler and more durable devices for measuring intraocular pressure are also needed.
6. Iridotomy should be the preferred treatment for angle-closure glaucoma. A simple, cheap, portable laser should be developed to permit this operation to be carried out in non-hospital settings.
7. Open-angle glaucoma should be treated only by medical means, if possible. However, when medical treatment proves ineffective or cannot be continued, surgery may be the treatment of choice.

OCULAR TRAUMA

Definition

World-wide, there are few statistics available on the incidence of blindness and visual loss caused by ocular trauma, or eye injury. However, studies in developing nations, as well as statistics from the industrialized countries, indicate that visual loss from eye injuries may be more prevalent than generally recognized. For example, estimates from the United States indicate that 19 400 people are blind because of eye injuries and an additional million have some degree of visual impairment from this cause.

Eye injuries occur in industrial settings, in schools, in sports activities, and when working in and around the home. In the United States, 300 000 eye injuries occur each year in the industrial sector, 95 000 in schools, and 40 000 in sports. In all countries, certain age and work groups appear more vulnerable than others to ocular accidents. For example, schoolchildren are the age group most likely to suffer eye injury. Among occupational groups, farmers tend to be at particular risk.

Protective eyewear can prevent or greatly reduce the seriousness of eye injuries. When ocular injury does occur, permanent visual loss usually can be avoided if the victim promptly obtains skilled medical care. Such care is widely available in countries with advanced medical services, for instance in the United States, where about 300 000 eye injuries are treated in hospital emergency rooms each year. Unfortunately, many people in the developing nations do not have access to the medical treatment needed to minimize visual damage from eye injuries. As a result, ocular trauma carries a much higher risk of visual loss in these nations than in the developed countries.

Problems and progress

A country's success in controlling eye injuries depends on the nature and extent of the ocular hazards its citizens are exposed to; on the scope and effectiveness of the efforts made by governmental agencies and other organizations to protect the eyes of workers, students, and the general public; and on the amount of progress made in developing eye safety educational programmes.

In the developed countries, large numbers of eye injuries continue to occur, despite the efforts that governments, industries, and schools have made to promote safety. Progress has been even more difficult in the developing nations, where efforts to reduce the toll of visual loss from ocular trauma have been hampered by a dearth of funds for public education programmes and shortages of medical personnel and facilities.

Strategy

Participants in the ocular trauma workshop at the Assembly recommended the following steps as part of any national campaign to prevent eye injuries:

1. Secure strong co-operation and participation of ophthalmology in prevention of eye injury by emphasizing this subject in training, residency, and ophthalmology society programmes.
2. Inform general physicians, occupational physicians, nurses, allied health personnel and teachers about eye protection and eye injury.
3. Conduct community educational campaigns using radio, television, newspapers and magazines to bring messages to the general public.
4. Create interest in eye safety programmes in government agencies such as the safety division of the labour department and the education, industrial, and health departments; and in community organizations such as Lions, Rotary, Red Cross, and organizations for the blind.
5. Secure government regulations requiring eye protection where needed.
6. Investigate methods of providing safety glasses (for example, through a contribution from an optical company).
7. Obtain other needed resources, such as:
    (a) materials for professional and public education programmes;
    (b) radio and television programmes on eye safety issues, including brief ('spot') announcements that can be broadcast repeatedly;
    (c) slide-tape presentations for physicians, nurses, and other professionals.
    (d) leaflets;
    (e) films; and
    (f) guides for schools and industry.
8. Conduct research on ocular trauma, including studies to determine the number, types, causes, and costs of eye injuries.

Dr Kupfer wishes to acknowledge the admirable source material for this chapter provided by the participants of the Assembly workshops under the chairmanship of Dr Dawson (trachoma), Dr Sommer (xerophthalmia), Professor Quarcoopome (onchocerciasis), Professor Nakajima (cataract), Dr Linner (glaucoma), and Dr Contreras (ocular trauma). He also wishes to acknowledge the invaluable information contained in the various publications resulting from the World Health Organization's Advisory Group on the Prevention of Blindness and from its specialized programmes.

3

Retrospect
Sir John Wilson

The formation of the International Agency for the Prevention of Blindness in January 1975 was the culmination of years of pioneer work by individuals and organizations. It marked also a new awareness of the scale and consequences of blindness in the developing countries and a growing recognition of the means by which much of that blindness could be avoided.

In its composition, The Agency expressed a partnership which had been developing in the previous decade between ophthalmic surgeons acting through their national and international organizations, and the organizations of and for the blind. To these organizations, with their humanitarian motivation and fund-raising capability, this represented a significant broadening of the role which they had previously conceived in terms of rehabilitation and welfare. Individual ophthalmic surgeons had done outstanding pioneer work, and organizations like the International Association for the Prevention of Blindness and the International Organization against Trachoma had been outstanding advocates of blindness prevention within the ophthalmic profession. However, for most ophthalmologists in traditional urban practices, the prospect of a global strategy against blindness presented a new professional dimension. The World Health Organization played its essential part in the creation of the Agency. In successive resolutions between 1969 and 1975, the World Health Assembly expanded its mandate from concern for two specific eye diseases—trachoma and onchocerciasis—into a programme concerned with the major causes of preventable blindness in developing countries. The procedure by which this expansion was achieved was an example of that interaction between private enterprises and government initiative, between specialized interests and general policy, which so often is the originating impulse of new international movements.

In 1972 the WHO convened a study group with a representative membership including people who, in various countries, had been advocating blindness prevention. One of the main recommendations of this committee, was for the establishment of an organization to co-ordinate non-governmental action and to mobilize international interest and resources for systematic action.

That was the beginning of a fruitful partnership between the WHO and the Agency. An inter-regional meeting in Baghdad played a large part in identifying objectives and priorities. Attention was focused on those countries which have an excessive prevalence of avoidable blindness (later defined as more than 1 per cent of the population) where the objective was to reduce that prevalence to the greatest practical extent. Four diseases were identified together accounting for most of the avoidable blindness in developing countries—onchocerciasis, trachoma, cataract, and xerophthalmia. These became the priorities both of the WHO and of the Agency but it is interesting to recall that there was much argument at the outset about the inclusion of cataract on the grounds that it was 'curable' not preventable. This was one direction in which the influence of the blind welfare organizations prevailed with their insistence that a programme of blindness prevention would lack immediacy and cutting edge unless one of its priorities was to restore sight to the curable blind.

The Agency early identified two additional priorities—glaucoma and ocular accident—and emphasized that its concern was also for the causes of avoidable blindness in industrialized countries. At the Agency's first general assembly in 1978, the link between blindness and ageing was emphasized with the prediction that, unless effective action was taken to break that link, the number of blind people in industrialized countries would be likely to double in the next 50 years. More recently, the emphasis has increasingly moved away from a 'disease orientated' strategy to a 'problem orientated' concept. Probably these are different stages to what has always been seen as the initial objective of attacking avoidable blindness from whatever cause everywhere.

The essential requirements of the strategy were action at the 'country level'. For the Agency this meant the formation of national committees. For WHO it meant the establishment of national programmes for the prevention of blindness. This was another area of effective collaboration because usually the adoption of a national programme by government was preceded by the establishment of a non-governmental committee with the ability to mobilize national interest and resources and to generate political will. The formation of these national committees was one of the Agency's priorities during its initial years and by the time of the Second General Assembly in Washington (1982) committees were in existence in 56 countries.

To facilitate collaboration with the WHO Regional Office, the Agency established regional committees in Africa, Eastern Europe, Latin America, the Middle East, North America, Southern Asia, Western Europe, and the Western Pacific.

In 1976, WHO adopted the prevention of blindness as one of the priorities of its global programme of technical co-operation. This lead was followed by the identification of blindness as a WHO regional priority in South-East Asia, the Eastern Mediterranean, Africa, and the Americas. Full-time advisers on the prevention of blindness have now been appointed in Africa and South-East Asia.

National programmes for the prevention of blindness followed first in Asia (where the Indian national programme marked a major step forward), and increasingly in other regions. At the meeting of WHO's

Advisory Group in 1983 it was reported that national programmes were in operation in 24 countries with the expectation that in five years there were likely to be national programmes in some 60 developing countries.

The WHO's Programme Advisory Group on the Prevention of Blindness, which has met annually since 1978, is another convincing demonstration of effective co-operation between UN agencies, governments, and non-governmental interests. It has given to this whole movement a definition and precision of planning which could not have been achieved in any other way. From it have come some admirable policy documents on statistics, economic justification, primary eye care, strategies, and the essential documentation on personnel training, research options, and clinical procedures. The Reports of the Meetings of this Advisory Group show a constant development of the programme.

One far-reaching development from this group meeting has been the establishment of WHO Collaborating Centres for the Prevention of Blindness. Twelve such centres now exist, primarily concerned with planning, research, and staff training. Others are being designated as the programme advances. Two of these Centres, in London and Baltimore, offer an international course in community eye care.

Amongst the strongest supporters of the global programme are the non-governmental organizations which are in official relationships with the WHO or are international members of the Agency. Amongst these are the International Federation of Ophthalmic Societies and the International Organization against Trachoma which operate within the ophthalmic profession, and the World Council for the Welfare of the Blind. Notable financial support has come from the international members of the Agency which include the Christoffel Blindenmission, Helen Keller International, the International Eye Foundation, Operation Eyesight Universal, the Seva Foundation and the Royal Commonwealth Society for the Blind. Largely as a result of these organizations the amount of non-governmental funding now exceeds $20 million annually.

With its Voluntary Funds for Health Promotion, the WHO has established a special account for the prevention of blindness. Substantial resources have been contributed to that fund notably by Japan, the Netherlands, Norway, the United States, and the Arab Gulf Programme for UN Development Organizations.

These are the main components of what has now become a global programme for the prevention of blindness. Its practical achievements are elaborated in this book. Much remains to be done, but much has been achieved not least in a significant expansion in our conceptual framework.

At the World Congress of Ophthalmology in San Francisco (1982) and at the meetings of the Regional Ophthalmic Academy, the prevention of blindness has been increasingly recognized as a new and essential international dimension in ophthalmology. Community eye care has become a priority of health policy and, with a distinct strategy and multidisciplinary staff, it is almost acquiring the status of a separate discipline.

These advances are part of a more general movement in international policies of health and development. The concept of 'Health for All by the Year 2000' which was promulgated at the Alma Ata conference and which has been adopted as its central aim by the WHO, has its obvious implication for 'eye health for all'. In the International Year of the Child, eye diseases such as trachoma and xerophthalmia were recognized as important contributors to childhood deprivation and UNICEF entered this field with its special commitment and enthusiasm. In the International Year of Disabled Persons (1981) and the Decade of Action which followed it, the prevention of disablement has been adopted as an essential objective and the prevention of blindness programme has been cited as the most convincing demonstration that such an objective is attainable.

October 1983, as this book goes to press, marks the inauguration of Impact, the international initiative against avoidable disablement promoted by the United Nations Development Programme, UNICEF, and WHO. It is no coincidence that this new and far-reaching international programme is benefiting, not only in its basic concepts and vocabulary, but also in the experience of its personnel from the international programme for the prevention of blindness.

4

Regional action

The International Agency for the Prevention of Blindness has nine Regional Committees for the Prevention of Blindness. The Chairmen of each of these Committees reported to the Second General Assembly on progress achieved within these regions during the four years elapsing since the First General Assembly was held in Oxford, England in 1978. Their reports follow.

AFRICA

Professor C. O. Quarcoopome reported that the Africa region lags behind all others in that none of the countries in the region is operating an identifiable blindness prevention programme. Kenya may be considered an exception as it has a limited programme. An identifiable national blindness prevention programme in Africa should be characterized by:

(a) being based on the results of a sound blindness prevalence survey;
(b) according priority consideration to the worst affected areas and the most common causes of avoidable blindness;
(c) being based, as far as possible, on the primary-health-care approach in order to ensure maximum coverage of the population;
(d) having an identifiable individual who will act as a national focal point and who will co-ordinate all prevention of blindness activities; and
(e) an operating budget.

The magnitude of the problem

The number of blind persons in Africa is not known with any accuracy, but it is estimated that the figure must be between 3.5 and 5 million. The problem is further compounded by the high rate of population growth. Furthermore, the estimate does not take into account the high morbidity due to severe visual impairment.

Ignorance, poverty, superstition, adverse cultural practices, and sometimes fatalistic indifference, contribute to the gravity of the problem in Africa.

It is clear the African region is facing many difficulties in its efforts to establish viable blindness prevention programmes. Among these, the deteriorating economic situation in almost all the countries is the most serious. Balance of payment difficulties and other factors are having an adverse effect on health budgets. In many countries there has been a deterioration in the health service provided. This has made investment in fresh areas and recruitment of necessary staff rather difficult.

It is necessary for all African governments to accept that basic eye care services must be funded from local sources if these services are to be durable. However, it may be appropriate for external assistance to be sought for the funding of specific time-limited studies, surveys or control activities.

The lack of data on the prevalence, causes, and distribution of blinding conditions urgently needs to be corrected to enable meaningful planning to be carried out. The real take-off of the blindness programme will be expedited when the data deficit has been eliminated. To this end a pool of consultants, willing and able to carry out prevalence and other surveys, should be established to provide assistance.

Major causes of blindness in Africa

The major blinding conditions in Africa are trachoma, onchocerciasis, nutritional blindness, glaucoma, and trauma, while the magnitude of the problem of cataract in Africa is only now being realized. These major causes mask the minor ones such as congenital, developmental or genetic defects, diabetes and sickle cell disease, uveitis and a whole range of retinal degenerations, and optic atrophies.

The population of Africa is comparatively young and it is to be expected that with an increasing life-span the degenerative eye diseases will add their toll to the existing causes of blindness.

The geographical distribution of blindness

Onchocerciasis is found in most of the countries of Africa between latitudes 15°N and 15°S. The worst areas for blindness are the savannah zones.

Trachoma is endemic in the Sahelian belt and the Sudan as well as many countries in Central and Southern Africa.

Blindness from cataract is common throughout Africa and is recognized as a major problem in early middle age and often in younger persons.

Nutritional blindness is widespread in the Sahelian areas and in East, Central, and Southern Africa. Curiously, many countries in West Africa do not consider xerophthalmia as a serious public health problem. But this must be viewed with caution because many cases may be subclinical.

Open-angle glaucoma is found in all countries but acute closed angle glaucoma is said to be uncommon. Many workers in the field think that surgery should be the first choice in the treatment of glaucoma in Africa.

Progress in prevention of blindness activities

The adoption of resolution R18, in relation to the programme for the prevention of blindness in Africa by the thirtieth session of the

World Health Organization Regional Committee for Africa in 1980, is the most significant event of the quadrennium under review. By this resolution all the African governments recognized the importance of blindness as a priority health problem, and undertook to take appropriate action towards its prevention. The resolution gave a regional policy basis to the blindness prevention programme.

The Onchocerciasis Control Programme of the Volta River Basin area has progressed satisfactorily, and has succeeded in achieving virtual control of the vector black-fly in 80 per cent of the programme area of about 750 000 sq km. Evaluation has shown that children under the age of 5 years no longer suffer from onchocerciasis, and that the prevalence rates of the disease have been reduced considerably. Studies have been undertaken regarding the feasibility of extending the programme area to Guinea-Bissau, Nigeria, Senegal, and The Gambia. Several onchocercal endemic countries are carrying out epidemiological surveys to determine the extent of the disease in order to assess its public health importance.

The African Regional Office of the WHO (AFRO) now has a part-time officer responsible for the prevention of blindness programme. The officer's other duties have previously tended to place blindness prevention in a subordinate position.

Since the 1980 Regional Committee resolution on blindness prevention, AFRO has despatched short-term consultants to several African countries to study and advise on the magnitude of the problem and the development of national programmes. Among the countries which have benefited are Botswana, Ethiopia, The Gambia, Ghana, Lesotho, Liberia, Malawi, Sierra Leone, Sudan, Swaziland, Togo, Zambia, and Zimbabwe. Moreover, a WHO-sponsored multinational workshop was recently held in Accra, Ghana to develop a national programme. There were participants from The Gambia, Ghana, Nigeria, and Sierra Leone.

A number of voluntary organizations have contributed significantly to prevention of blindness programmes; these include the following.

(1) *The International Eye Foundation* has been carrying out blindness prevention programmes, including the training of ophthalmic clinical assistants in Kenya, for many years with considerable success. Some of the assistants are trained in performing cataract surgery and are a commendable asset to the country. In collaboration with the WHO the Foundation sponsored a workshop in Bamako, Mali, in February 1979, to formulate guidelines for the planning of national and regional programmes for the prevention of blindness in Africa, and for ophthalmologists interested in blindness prevention to share experiences. Nine African countries, both English and French speaking, were represented. Another prevention of blindness meeting was held in Lilongwe, Malawi.

(2) *The Royal Commonwealth Society for the Blind* has maintained its active collaboration with several countries of the British Commonwealth and has been assisting with mobile clinics and personnel.
(3) *The International Vitamin A Consultative Group* has extended special interest and activity within Africa. With the assistance of the United States Agency for International Development programme (USAID) and the collaboration of the WHO it has sponsored studies on nutritional blindness in several African countries and organized a meeting in Nairobi, Kenya, in November 1981 to discuss and highlight the vitamin-A problem in Africa.

Summary of country activities

With over 50 countries in Africa it is not feasible to present a country-by-country report. Moreover, information from many of the countries is not available at present. Brief details are given below from selected countries.

Botswana

The population of Botswana is estimated to be 884 000 (1981). The prevalence of blindness is not known but is expected to be approximately 1.5 per cent on the basis of studies of comparable geographic, climatic, and socio-economic areas of Kenya. Cataract (40 per cent), trachoma (20 per cent), glaucoma (15 per cent), and trauma (9 per cent) are the prime causes of blindness as shown from hospital statistics. The two ophthalmologists on short-term contracts in the country are inadequately utilized due to lack of facilities and support staff. A WHO short-term consultant has made proposals for the training and better utilization of ophthalmic auxiliaries.

Ghana

In a population of about 12 million (1982) there are between 70 000 and 100 000 blind persons. Fifteen ophthalmologists operate between them static eye care services in nine centres and one mobile clinic. The National Committee for the Prevention of Blindness, formed in 1976, is being revived to spearhead a revitalized programme. A national co-ordinator has been appointed. A draft document for a national programme has been prepared by a WHO short-term consultant, while a workshop on the subject was sponsored by the World Health Organization together with the Government of Ghana. The workshop was attended by participants from Nigeria, The Gambia, and Sierra Leone. This novel approach to the preparation of a national prevention of blindness programme proved to be very useful, and should be studied by other countries. The Onchocerciasis Control Programme has yielded extremely satisfactory results in northern Ghana.

Kenya

Kenya has a population of 19 million, and the country has maintained its high awareness of and activities against blindness. It has static eye care clinics and a well organized mobile ophthalmic service. Kenya has an ongoing blindness prevention programme, and has shown the value and effectiveness of the use of ophthalmic clinical officers (ophthalmic medical assistants) in the delivery of eye care services. The rural eye care service provided with the assistance of the International Eye Foundation is a lesson that all African countries could usefully learn.

Lesotho

This country has a population of 1.33 million. Cataract, glaucoma, and corneal opacification are the major causes of blindness. In a 1982 study a prevalence of blindness of 1.23 per cent was reported, but limitations to the estimate's reliability due to sample design were commented on. There are four ophthalmologists in Lesotho, three of whom are expatriates. Proposals have been made for the development of a national prevention of blindness programme.

Liberia, The Gambia, and Sierra Leone

These three West African countries have each appointed a person to act as a national focal point for the development of a national prevention of blindness programme. Liberia has shown a high awareness of the problem of blindness and has contact with Operation Eyesight Universal of Canada in the development of eye care services. The programme is rather urban oriented and has had less than the desired impact on the problem of blindness. The shortage of trained personnel is a considerable obstacle. Sierra Leone has a serious onchocerciasis problem and in areas without this disease cataract, glaucoma, and trauma are the principal blinding conditions. The Gambia is not yet sufficiently aware of the problem of blindness in its population. These three countries have had the benefit of a WHO short-term consultant to stimulate the development of national prevention of blindness programmes.

Malawi

The country-wide prevalent of blindness in the population of 6 million people is not yet known. Surveys and studies have been carried out during the past four years. Cataract is the commonest cause of blindness (40 per cent). Trachoma (15 per cent) is found in the Lower Shire Valley. Corneal blindness/avitaminosis A associated with measles (15 per cent) is country-wide but is particularly prevalent in the Lower Shire Valley. The WHO Expanded Programme on Immunization which started in Malawi in 1978, appears to have decreased the incidence of corneal blindness due to measles in children. Glaucoma, estimated at 8 per cent is country-wide and onchocerciasis at 2 per cent is found in the Thylo district. The cataract problem is recognized as requiring urgent attention because, with only two ophthalmologists and one ophthalmic clinical assistant currently performing cataract surgery, the estimated backlog of at least 24 000 cases will continue to increase. Health services in Malawi are restricted by lack of resources in trained health personnel and a lack of adequate funds to meet the cost of salaries, equipment, supplies, transport, and the maintenance and repair of equipment and facilities. Most of the resources go to support central and district hospital curative services. A primary health care programme has started and is expected to provide eye care. Ophthalmic medical assistants are being trained, but training in intraocular surgery is not being carried out owing to lack of facilities and equipment. Far-reaching recommendations have been made by a short-term consultant.

Mali

There are 1.2 million people suffering from trachoma in Mali, while onchocerciasis is hyperendemic and blindness from the disease is widespread. Cataract is a major cause of blindness even in the 30 to 50 year age group. Glaucoma and hypovitaminosis A are other serious causes of blindness. Epidemiological studies have been carried out and Operation YELEEN (Operation Light) has been developed as a programme of mobile clinics and rural eye care to bring 'light' to those who are blind, and to prevent blindness in Mali. The campaign, started in 1979 for an initial four-year period (now extended by two years), will eventually be integrated into the government's health service.

Swaziland

The estimated population of Swaziland is 566 000 (1981). It has a peculiar rural settlement consisting of extended family homesteads; 14 per cent of these having no resident adult male and 83 per cent having an absentee male. The males are working abroad. The leading causes of visual loss are cataract, trauma, glaucoma, corneal disease, and uveitis. Trachoma has been found among schoolchildren and deserves further study. There are 52 doctors in Swaziland. The single ophthalmologist is an expatriate. No Swazi ophthalmologists have been trained or are in the process of being trained. The prevalence of blindness is not known and there is no current prevention of blindness programme.

Togo

The prevalence of blindness for the whole country (estimated population of 2.5 million) is not known. Surveys have shown a variation in different areas from 1 to 4 per cent. Onchocerciasis exists in the whole country, trachoma is present but its importance needs to be studied, and cataract is a problem from the age of 40 years. There are 121 physicians (1979), 94 medical assistants (1981) and five ophthalmic nurses. There is no ongoing prevention of blindness programme but surveys are being carried out.

Zambia

The population is estimated to be 6 million. The national prevalence of blindness is determined at 1.42 per cent, with a national prevalence of low vision (less than 6/18 or 0.3) of 3 per cent. The major causes of blindness in Zambia are cataract (30 per cent), trachoma (20 per cent), glaucoma (7 per cent), corneal disease (8 per cent), nutritional/ measles (5 per cent), trauma (5 per cent), and degenerative disease (15 per cent). The volume of cataract surgery carried out in Zambia is inadequate. Ophthalmologists are mostly concentrated in the urban areas handling minor complaints because of the lack of hospital and operating time which would be necessary to accommodate major surgical patients. There are 689 doctors in Zambia with 17 ophthalmologists (1981) and 1215 medical assistants. A mobile clinic unit is operating satisfactorily and a second one is due to be established in 1983.

Zimbabwe

In a population of 7.13 million (1979), the prevalence of blindness is 1.2 per cent with a prevalence of impaired vision of 3.7 per cent. Senile cataract is the leading cause of blindness (40 per cent). The estimated backlog of approximately 80 000 cases of cataract is certain to rise, as only three governmental ophthalmologists and two other doctors are performing cataract surgery. This is compounded by an exaggerated hospital stay due to distance from the patients' homes, lack of postoperative care other than in the Central Hospital, and loss of bed space due to injuries and other emergencies. There is a three-year waiting list for cataract surgery at the Harare Hospital Eye Unit. Trachoma (20 per cent) is an important cause of blindness, together with corneal blindness (10 per cent), glaucoma (10 per cent), trauma (4 per cent), and nutritional/blindness (1 per cent). Recommendations have been made for the development of a national prevention of blindness programme and a person to act as a national focal point has been appointed.

EASTERN EUROPE

Colonel Boris Zimin of the USSR, who was unable to attend the Assembly, provided reports on countries in the Eastern European region as described below. He emphasized the importance each country placed on prevention of blindness activities through the state systems of public health services. However, new questions are arising which may only be resolved by co-ordinating activities between countries. The Unions of the Blind in Bulgaria, Hungary, Rumania, and the USSR are considering holding a regional symposium during 1983-4 to bring together experts on the prevention of blindness and on medical and social rehabilitation of visually handicapped people in Eastern Europe.

The Soviet Union

Eye care and prevention of blindness work is organized as one of the most important activities of public health and social welfare services of the country. A free ophthalmological service is made available through various state and social measures regulated by state decrees. This includes the prevention of eye diseases and trauma, and medical and social rehabilitation of visually impaired people. Prevention of blindness programmes are based on a detailed systematic study of the various causes of blindness and instances of eye diseases in different regions of the country.

Thanks to comprehensive medical care, the extent of blindness has been more than halved; while blindness as a result of trachoma, smallpox, venereal, and other social diseases, has been eradicated from the country. The principal causes of visual impairment are currently atrophy of the optic nerve, glaucoma, severe myopia, retinal disorders, and lens diseases.

Ophthalmological services are provided through a wide range of eye clinics, eye diseases departments of hospitals, laboratories, poly-clinics, and medical care departments at industrial enterprises. Specialized centres of eye microsurgery, ophthalmic traumatology, ophthalmic oncology, laser surgery, anti-glaucoma, and contact lens centres, and medical and social rehabilitation centres for the visually impaired are found throughout the country.

Ophthalmological services are based on regular dispensary examinations of those patients suffering from the most dangerous eye diseases, for example glaucoma, severe myopia, and optic nerve pathology, as well as from other visual impairments. The whole population is regularly examined by eye doctors for early diagnosis of glaucoma and other eye diseases.

Great importance is attached to the care of children's sight. A special ophthalmological service with a wide range of children's eye clinics, eye-care centres, and sanatoria has been set up. Ophthalmological examinations are available to all children from birth, with dispensary check-ups for all children with myopia, strabismus, amblyopia, glaucoma, retinal diseases, etc.

Scientific research is conducted in accordance with state programmes of research and development in the field of ophthalmology and prevention of blindness. Research institutions of ophthalmology as well as eye disease departments of medical institutes and universities have successfully developed eye microsurgery, and optic-reconstructive operations, including artificial lens implantation and keratoprosthesis. Good results are achieved in early diagnosis and treatment of glaucoma, myopia, virus eye diseases, pathology of the retina, etc. Laser ophthalmological surgery is now also under development.

Close contacts between research and health care institutions contribute to a better realization of scientific achievements and to the improvement of ophthalmological services. Press, radio, and television are widely used in prevention work.

All activities on prevention of blindness and especially on rehabilitation of visually impaired people are arranged in close contact with associations of the blind throughout the country, the leader in this field being the All-Russia Association of the Blind. A scientifically based system of medical and social rehabilitation of the visually impaired has been created. This includes a complex of medical, psychological, social, pedagogical, and vocational programmes aimed at complete rehabilitation and social integration of visually impaired people. To co-ordinate the various activities in the field the All-Russia Union and the Union Republics' Committees on Prevention of Blindness have been formed.

The USSR shares its experience with other countries, and helps some of them in their struggle against blindness. Mostly this experience is used in socialist countries, where both the state and social activities are aimed at the development and the improvement of ophthalmological services and the prevention of blindness.

Editor's note. An interesting sidelight on the relationship within the Soviet Union between organizations of the blind and the ophthalmic profession is that, during the past 15 years, approximately $75 million, being part of the profits made by employment and other enterprises for the blind, have been used to build 14 major eye hospitals and to promote ophthalmic research.

Bulgaria

A National Committee on Prevention of Blindness has been founded with ophthalmologists, representatives of the Union of the Blind, and members of other social organizations forming the committee. Within the prevention of blindness programmes considerable importance has been given to the epidemiological study of blindness to identify all those who are visually impaired so that they may have the social and vocational rehabilitation services they need, including regular dispensary check-ups.

Epidemiological studies of blindness have demonstrated the benefits of active prevention and medical measures which have considerably reduced the number of cases of blindness caused by glaucoma, industrial accidents, and infectious eye diseases. The structure of blindness has been shown to have changed, the main causes of blindness now are inborn and hereditary eye diseases, eye trauma, inflammatory diseases, and retinal disorders, associated with systemic diseases or ageing (e.g. diabetic retinopathy and senile macular degeneration).

Improvements in the early diagnosis of eye diseases are constantly being made together with advances in a range of treatments including eye microsurgery and laser surgery.

A scheme to provide gainful employment for visually handicapped people, based on the principles of the USSR system, has been developed.

Czechoslovakia

Preventive measures have helped to eliminate such causes of blindness as trachoma and venereal diseases, and blindness caused by eye trauma has been reduced. The most complicated problems in the field at present are the prevention and cure of retrolental fibroplasia, pigmentary degeneration of the retina, and diabetic retinopathy. Successful research in the field of genetics is playing an important role in combatting these problems.

German Democratic Republic

The main causes of blindness are glaucoma, severe myopia, senile macular degeneration, cataract, and eye trauma. Thanks to an active programme including dispensary check-ups and other measures, blindness caused by glaucoma and diabetes has been reduced.

The national mass media and special services on safety at work are used to popularize measures designed to reduce the incidence of ocular trauma in industrial settings and in everyday life.

Hungary

Blindness caused by trachoma and venereal diseases has been eradicated. The main causes of blindness now are glaucoma, vascular disorders of the retina, diabetes, inflammatory and viral diseases of the cornea and uveal tract, cataract, eye trauma, and retrolental fibroplasia.

Preventive measures are aimed first at an early diagnosis of glaucoma. For this purpose the whole population over 40 years of age is regularly examined by eye doctors. Genetic consultations are arranged in order to prevent hereditary eye diseases. These consultations are especially important when blind couples are deciding whether to have children. Great importance is attached to the care of children's sight and the early diagnosis of amblyopia and strabismus.

Methods of early diagnosis and curing of eye diseases are constantly improving, particularly in the field of laser ophthalmology.

Rumania

Medical and social programmes on the national level are aimed at the prevention of blindness, early diagnosis of eye diseases, improvement of the ophthalmological service, and social and vocational rehabilitation of the visually impaired. The main causes of blindness are glaucoma, pigmentary degeneration of the retina, congenital and hereditary eye diseases, macular degeneration, hypertensive retinopathy, myopia, and chronic infectious diseases of the uveal tract. The total population, especially children between five and seven years of age, and those undergoing vocational assessment courses or changing employment have ophthalmological examinations. Considerable attention is given to hygienic and well-planned working conditions in order to minimize the incidence of eye trauma.

Children with myopia and strabismus receive regular examinations and treatment at dispensaries. While early diagnosis and examinations are also provided for patients with glaucoma in regional hospitals and ophthalmic clinics. Optic-reconstructive operations (lens extraction at high myopia, implantation of artificial lens, transplantation of cornea) and correction of refractive errors by means of contact lenses are increaasingly being developed.

As a result of all these measures, the number of visually impaired people in Rumania has been considerably reduced during the last five years. Programmes have also been arranged in the field of social and vocational rehabilitation with emphasis on integration, vocational training, and gainful employment.

Yugoslavia

The main causes of blindness are inborn and hereditary diseases and eye trauma. Work on prevention of blindness involves close collaboration of research and medical and pedagogical institutes and social organizations.

The eye care of the population is one of the most important activities of the public health services and is provided free. Regular ophthalmological examinations of all children from birth to 7 years is compulsory and dispensary treatment is organized for those who are found to have visual impairment. The operational efficiency of the ophthalmological service through its delivery of eye care to the general public is constantly improving, with an expansion of medical institutions and staff training and the development of scientific ophthalmological research. In addition, considerable attention is given to the basic medical education of the population in the field of eye care and the prevention of eye trauma in industry and everyday life. Thanks to these measures the number of blind people in Yugoslavia is steadily decreasing.

LATIN AMERICA

Dr Francisco Contreras Campos of Peru reported that Multi-Disciplinary National Committees have been formed to execute programmes for the prevention of blindness. Coverage and intensity are variable, but all are fully aware of the need to reduce the number of cases of avoidable blindness. An important activity is the evaluation of the major causes of ocular diseases in the countries of Latin America. At the same time a general plan has been established to co-ordinate activities throughout the area.

Latin America comprises a group of nations that can be identified under similar cultural, socio-economic, and geographic features within the international sphere. Nevertheless, every one of the countries possesses different characteristics that contribute to the development of appropriate programmes for the preventionof blindness according to need.

Ocular disorders have been traditionally approached in Latin America from the therapeutic point of view. Also, there has been an overwhelming urban distribution of ophthalmologists. At the present time, ophthalmologists are becoming more conscious of the significance of prevention, as well as the need for multisectoral collaboration to carry out the activities necessary to bring about a reduction of avoidable blindness.

The Organizacion Panamericana de la Salud in collaboration with other institutions has organized two regional seminars and two subregional seminars devoted to the evaluation of the prevention of blindness programmes within the Latin American environment. Although as yet no statistical studies have been undertaken, the importance accorded to the subject is evident from the interest aroused in the various countries of the region.

Brief details of various countries' programmes are given below.

Brazil

A World Health Organization Collaborating Centre for the Prevention of Blindness has been established. This Centre is developing a National Programme for Eye Care in collaboration with the Ministry of Health.

Caribbean

Barbados is trying to co-ordinate training activities for physicians and auxiliary personnel in ocular assistance that may be of benefit to all the countries in the Caribbean.

Chile

Glaucoma screening has been undertaken together with campaigns for the prevention of domestic and industrial ocular accidents. Activities for the prevention of amblyopia and ocular accidents are also under way. These programmes are being carried out under the aegis of the Prevention of Blindness of the Sociedad Chilena de Oftalmologia and the Institute of Prevention of Blindness, who are now also working on a national survey concerned with the causes of blindness.

Colombia

There are various campaigns for the prevention of blindness co-ordinated by the Ministries of Health, Education, The Sociedad Colombiana de Oftalmologia, and the Instituto Nacional de Ciegos.

Costa Rica

Official organizations and universities are actively collaborating to prepare statistical data at national level on ocular diseases.

Guatemala

Training for prevention of blindness personnel at primary, secondary, and tertiary levels has priority in the Guatemalan Programme of the National Committee for the Blind. Research projects on trachoma, xerophthalmia, and onchocerciasis are being undertaken continuously.

The Institute of Visual Sciences was created in 1982, within the Medical Division of the National Committee for the Blind of Guatemala to co-ordinate training and research. The Dr Rodolfo Robles Hospital, as a World Health Organization Collaborating Centre, together with its rural centres, provides ophthalmic attention to 12 000 people a month.

Haiti

A separate report on Haiti was provided by Dr Reynold Monsanto, President of Eye Care Haiti who reported that of the 6 million Haitians 70 to 80 per cent live in rural areas while 80 per cent are illiterate. The government has two eye clinics—one at the University General Hospital in Port-au-Prince and the other in Cap-Haitien in the northern part of the island. Two other government clinics, less well equipped are situated in Les Cayes and St. Max. In the south of the country, Operation Eyesight Universal of Canada is also conducting a prevention of blindness campaign.

Since 1974, Helen Keller International has been working with the Government of Haiti's Bureau of Nutrition in a national programme to prevent nutritional blindness in children.

Eye Car Haiti (ECH) is a non-profit-making local organization dedicated to neglected vision. It operates five eye clinics in various parts of Haiti, in some of which there are facilities for performing operations. In two of the clinics ECH has trained two groups of nine young people from the community to work as ophthalmic assistants.

They receive a 1-year-training programme in which they learn to carry out a wide range of administrative and paramedical activities including routine tests.

ECH is concerned to reach as many people as possible in rural areas and to refer them to clinics attended by an ophthalmologist, where this is necessary. At the same time ECH carries out the education programmes for the general population and visits schools to test visual acuity.

ECH also promotes education amongst doctors providing them with library, lecturing, and other facilities. Young doctors on completion of their training may be offered a standing eye clinic where ECH provides drugs and equipment while the Government pays the doctor's salary.

ECH having undertaken a prevalence survey in one area is keen to proceed, when funds permit, to carry out further surveys and to use the knowledge as a basis for providing appropriate services.

Mexico

In Mexico there is a long established Instituto de Prevencion de Ceguera which has a charity ophthalmological clinic for people on low incomes living in the area. The Institute now intends to spread its activities to other parts of the country.

Peru

Training programmes are being provided for promoters who work in various rural areas of the country. This training forms part of the Primary Health Care Programme. Training is also provided for elementary schoolteachers in the detection of early ocular diseases in schoolchildren within the First Level. The work is co-ordinated by govermental and non-governmental, national and international organizations. The possibility of supplying low-cost spectacles to individuals of limited economic resources is being studied. These programmes are financed by Operation Eyesight Universal, Canada and also more recently by Helen Keller International.

Venezuela

The Venezuela Association for the Prevention of Blindness is actively collaborating with the Ministry of Health and Education and the Institute of Social Security to carry out campaigns to promote visual health for children and the prevention of accidents at work, as well as undertaking training courses for medical and paramedical personnel.

THE MIDDLE EAST

Sheikh Abdullah M. Al-Ghanim reported that it was not possible to make an accurate estimate of the number of blind people in the Middle East region, because of lack of information, and because each country defines blindness in relation to its own social and economic conditions. Therefore, the magnitude of the problem is not known in detail. However, the total number of blind people in the area is roughly estimated at 7.5 million (according to the report of the WHO Regional Committee in 1975). This represents an overall regional prevalence rate of about 3 per cent. Most of this blindness is the result of communicable diseases, notably trachoma and the acute ophthalmias.

A blindness rate of between 4.1 and 4.7 per cent has been regularly found in the trachoma-endemic areas of many countries in the region, for example Jordan, Egypt, Sudan, and Syria. The same high prevalence rate of blindness, 4.1 per cent, was observed in the trachoma-endemic area of Morocco. Of course, in areas free from endemic trachoma and other eye infections, the prevalence of blindness is much less. According to available data, the blindness rate may vary from 0.86 per cent in rural areas to 4.2 per cent in the urban areas of badly affected countries.

A specific and somewhat localized blindness problem is faced in areas where onchocerciasis and trachoma are endemic. This is a widespread and significant problem in Sudan, where approximately a million people are thought to be afflicted with these diseases, particularly in Bahr El-Ghazal and the Equatorial provinces. The prevalence rate of blindness in these parts of the Sudan is estimated at 5.1 per cent of which 4.9 per cent is due to onchocerciasis. A more localized and less severe onchocerciasis problem is prevalent in the Yemen Arab Republic.

In the Kingdom of Saudi Arabia there are, so far, no accurate or official statistics of blindness. However, according to some local investigations in hospitals and to special studies, the estimated prevalence rate of blindness in the Kingdom is 2 per cent. In a population of approximately 7 million people are about 140 000 blind.

Although great efforts have been exerted by most countries within the region to tackle the problem of blindness, nevertheless difficulties remain acute and severe. This may be attributable to the following reasons:

(a) delay of ophthalmological attention and care for patients suffering from eye diseases;
(b) lack of a practical programme for prevention of blindness as well as a national policy for the control of communicable eye diseases;
(c) lack of skilled medical manpower;
(d) lack of accurate and up-to-date statistics; and

(e) lack of specialized ophthalmological services especially in the rural areas.

Major causes of blindness in the region

The principal causes of blindness in the Middle East region are trachoma and other inflammations (mainly bacterial). About 150 million people are susceptible to eye diseases, especially trachoma, if proper preventive and curative measures are not taken. It has been found that more than 60 per cent of cases of blindness associated with these diseases could have been prevented by good hygiene and early treatment. The majority of preventable cases concern children.

One of the main factors affecting the prevalence of blindness is the high rate of allergic conjunctivitis in some countries such as the Kingdom of Saudi Arabia. In some areas, corneal ulcer is one of the most serious eye diseases. Other cases of blindness in the region are attributed to accidents, cataract, glaucoma, onchocerciasis, and errors of refraction.

One must state that, although no clear information or definite data are yet available, all concerned agree that eye diseases are one of the major health problems in the countries of the region and that the eye health care system in most of these countries is inadequate to meet the magnitude and complexities of the problem.

Progress in blindness prevention activities

The Regional Bureau of the Middle East Committee for the Blind has continued intensive efforts to adopt all preventive means and measures for the elimination of the causes of blindness, with particular emphasis on the control of blinding eye diseases in an effort to restrict the ceaseless increase of visual handicap in this region.

A summary of activities in which the Bureau has been involved follows.

1. The Bureau has adopted the idea of establishing a Regional Centre for the Prevention of Blindness with the aims of controlling eye diseases in the region and preventing blindness.
2. The Sixth Conference of the Gulf Arab States Ministries of Health was held in Muscat, Oman, in January 1979. In response to a memorandum on trachoma and the control of blindness in the area it was resolved that the Secretary-General of the Health Secretariat General for the Arab Countries of the Gulf Area, in collaboration with the Regional Bureau, should be empowered to set up a technical committee of ophthalmologists and prevention experts for studying the preventive, curative, and rehabilitative problems related to eye diseases.

3. This technical committee has made a number of resolutions and recommendations, significantly:
   (a) The establishment of an ophthalmic unit affiliated to the General Directorate of preventive medicine in each Ministry of Health in the Gulf Arab States. The units would develop programmes for the prevention of blindness and the control of communicable eye diseases.
   (b) The formulation of an advisory ophthalmic committee, with technical representatives from every member state which will be affiliated to the Health General Secretariat.

   The committee has held four meetings and among its resolutions and recommendations are the following:
   (i) to consider evaluation of the magnitude of the eye problems in each state by suitable methods;
   (ii) to prepare a comprehensive, informative and cultural programme in the field of eye hygiene;
   (iii) to consider the importance of training programmes for ophthalmologists and auxiliary personnel.
4. A number of awareness campaigns have been launched notably during the International Year of the Child (IYC) 1979 and the International Year of Disabled Persons (IYDP) 1981. In addition, the Bureau has issued a wide variety of educational materials and articles.
5. The Kingdom of Saudi Arabia has recently established a large specialized eye hospital with 265 beds in Riyadh City. The hospital is fully equipped with the most sophisticated equipment and modern medical apparatus, and is under the supervision of leading ophthalmologists and specialists.

   At the request and suggestion of the Bureau, a Regional Training and Research Centre, concerned with the prevention of blindness will be established inside the hospital campus with a view to serving the Arab Gulf States.
6. The Bureau has paid increasing attention to the needs of those with low vision and partial sight, considering this an important aspect of the prevention of blindness services. Countries within the region have been encouraged to introduce appropriate services through the establishment of specialized clinics within their health programmes. These clinics will be supervised by ophthalmologists and supplied with a staff of optometrists and opticians.

Egypt

To determine the rates and causes of visual loss in rural areas where 60 per cent of the Egyptian population lives, Professor Korra, Dr C. Dawson, and others (at the University of Alexandria, Egypt and Francis I. Proctor Foundation, University of California, San Francisco, USA) carried out a sample survey in 1979 and 1980. The survey utilized the new criteria and techniques set forth by the WHO programme for the prevention of blindness. The results of this survey are intended as a basis for devising more effective ways to deal with excessive blindness in Egypt. The prevalence of blindness in rural areas was found to be 1.8 per cent (1.6 per cent of males and 2 per cent of females).

Trachoma is still highly prevalent in the rural population with a peak prevalence among children between two and six years of age. Cataract is the primary cause of blindness (29 per cent), followed by trachoma complicated by acute ophthalmia (26 per cent), corneal opacity found in association with cataract (18 per cent), glaucoma (16 per cent), and other causes (10 per cent).

Measures are taken to treat those cataract patients who are supposed to be potentially blind, and to prevent trachoma and other eye infections in the rural areas.

Prevention of blindness programmes in Egypt are carried out mainly by the government. The Ministry of Public Health has more than 300 hospitals with ophthalmic departments and these are distributed throughout the country. These hospitals are well equipped, well staffed, and all the treatment is free, including operations and investigations. Between 2 and 3 million new cases are received each year mostly of acute ophthalmias, cataract, and glaucoma. In addition, all the universities have ophthalmic departments, where the population is given free treatment. The educational aspects of the programme are undertaken by the Egyptian Society for the Prevention of Blindness.

Jordan

An ophthalmological and social study of 137 blind and visually impaired students of the Al Nur Institute in Ashrafieh and the Regional Centre for Blindness in Shmesani, undertaken by Sayegh, Khoury, and Arafat, found the causes of blindness to be congenital in 79 per cent of cases and acquired in 21 per cent. The most common causes of congenital blindness were retinitis pigmentosa (23 per cent) and cataracts (17 per cent). The most common causes of acquired blindness were ocular infection (15 per cent) and injury (4 per cent). Genetic factors were shown to be the main causes of blindness: the rate of marriage between first cousins was 65 per cent among the parents of congenitally blind students, whereas the rate in the general population was 39 per cent.

Trachoma has been a serious problem in Jordan. In 1940 investigations by the WHO showed that 95 per cent of the population were affected. However, the introduction of trachoma prophylaxis by the Ministry of Health and the improvement of general living standards have reduced the incidence markedly. During the last 5 years only a few cases of active trachoma have been detected at the Jordan University Hospital in Amman.

Approval has been granted by the Ministry of Health for the setting up of a Jordanian Committee for the Prevention of Blindness. In addition, a mobile clinic is being brought into operation and an Ophthalmic Centre is to be established. The Centre will be responsible for prevention of blindness activities, treatment of patients, and rehabilitation of visually impaired and blind persons, as well as the medical care of blind and mentally retarded patients. Attachment to the University of Jordan will add teaching and research responsibilities to the Centre's programme.

Technical and financial support is needed to carry through this work. Support is also needed for the preparation of programmes for community-oriented teaching and for nursing and pre- and post-graduate studies in ophthalmology.

Pakistan

In a population of 90 million, 2 million people are blind and 20 million are visually impaired. The main causes of blindness are cataract, communicable eye disease, glaucoma, and injury. A national plan has been drawn up in which representatives from the community, social welfare and other voluntary organizations, and international voluntary agencies will co-operate with the Government of Pakistan to implement prevention of blindness activities and to provide eye care services throughout the country.

Through the Eye Camp Programme over 250 000 patients have been treated and over 15 000 cataract operations have been performed with the help of voluntary agencies and the Royal Commonwealth Society for the Blind.

There are 12 medical schools with ophthalmic departments and all 56 districts have specialists in government hospitals with prevention of blindness programmes where eye diseases are treated free of charge. In addition, the WHO has initiated the first training programme for ophthalmic assistants in Karachi.

Yemen

Activities are limited to individual treatment either medically or surgically, education of a small number of medical assistants, and the health education of the population. No survey has been carried out up to the end of 1982.

NORTH AMERICA

As Acting Regional Chairman for North America, Mrs Virgina Boyce reported on prevention of blindness activities in Canada and the United States for the period 1981-2.

Canada and the United States comprise the North America region. In both countries, programme planning and development are based on data showing the prevalence and incidence of eye diseases, causes of blindness, and age and geographic distributions. In Canada, there are approximately 50 000 blind people, in the United States about 500 000. The leading causes of blindness in North America are glaucoma, macular degeneration, cataract, optic nerve atrophy, diabetes, and congenital and hereditary eye diseases. Diabetes is the leading cause of new cases of blindness in people between the ages of 20 and 74. The preventable causes of visual impairment are glaucoma, cataract, and trauma. There is good promise that blindness from diabetic retinopathy and macular degeneration will be reduced with new treatment methods.

The programmes of the Canadian National Institute for the Blind and the United States National Society to Prevent Blindness encompass public and professional education, community services, and research.

Canada

Since the First General Assembly of IAPB the Canadian National Institute for the Blind (CNIB), ophthalmologists and other disciplines in Canada have continued to stress the need for prevention of blindness. The following are same of the main activities undertaken.

1. Educational campaigns have been intensified to alert the public to the need for eye protection at home, in sports, and at play.
2. The Wise Owl Eye Safety Incentive Programme has continued to promote the wearing of eye protection in industry.
3. The need for rubella immunization has been stressed. Two of the provinces now have laws stating that a child must be vaccinated before entering school.
4. Seminars on eye health, on eye disease interpretation and prevention, and eye safety for professionals in the health field have been held across the country.
5. Workshops have been organized by the CNIB and ophthalmologists for general medical doctors to alert them to the need for early detection of glaucoma.
6. Courses on basic eye care and pre-school vision screening have been given to public health nurses.
7. The Eye Bank Programme has continued to function and expand across Canada.
8. Continuing eye care has been provided to underserved populations in northern, north-west, and Arctic regions through university departments of ophthalmology in these provinces. Care is delivered through air service and mobile units funded by CNIB and the Canadian Ministry of Health. This programme has created great

awareness of the need for early detection of eye trouble and the importance of regular eye care among public health nurses, family physicians, Lions, and other service clubs.

There has been increased activity in programmes concerned with the prevention of industrial eye injuries through a joint working relationship between the Construction Association and the Canadian Safety Council.

United States

The programme development of the National Society to Prevent Blindness is guided by advisory committees composed of ophthalmologists and other professionals. Their participation assures sound scientific direction.

The National Society, which serves the nation as a primary source of statistics on the prevalence and incidence of blinding eye diseases and other vision problems, completed important surveys on ocular injuries in schools, and a study of the vision standards for motor vehicle operators. Results of these studies indicate that more eye injuries occur in physical education classes, playgrounds, and classrooms than in laboratories and shops, and the motor vehicle operator licensing study disclosed that 12 states do not recheck drivers' vision when licences are renewed. Both of these studies provide important evidence on where the Society's programme activities should be concentrated.

In 1981, the National Society co-sponsored a conference on glaucoma together with the Japanese Glaucoma Research Society which was telecast by satellite. The team of experts in the United States shared their views with a panel of Japanese counterparts and an audience of 2000 professionals. Since then, over 10 000 physicians in Japan and the United States have seen the programme on videotape.

Glaucoma is still the nation's number one cause of preventable blindness and, as such, a major focus of the Society's efforts. As part of an extensive public education programme on glaucoma the Society's film, *Seeing*, which carries the message about the joys of sight and the value of early glaucoma detection has been seen by over 10 million people on television and in group showings. Two series of television spots about glaucoma are widely broadcast. Both were dubbed to reach the nation's Spanish-speaking population. The National Society has worked closely with the American Pharmaceutical Association to distribute information on the Society's glaucoma educational materials to the drug store customers. Screenings for glaucoma reach approximately 100 000 persons annually and are directed to increasing public knowledge about glaucoma.

As diabetic retinopathy is now the leading cause of new cases of blindness in adults, the National Society has prepared an exhibit and television announcements about the disease and the importance of regular eye examinations for every diabetic. In addition, the Society has introduced three educational tools for use with primary-care physicians and other health care professionals concerned with diagnosis and treatment of diabetic retinopathy: a scientific exhibit, a colour slide/tape presentation—*Diabetes and the eye*—and a brochure to establish its programme plan. To facilitate patient referral, the Society has published a listing of medical centres participating in clinical trials. The Society is also working closely with the American Academy of Family Physicians in distributing the programme on diabetic retinopathy.

The Society's recommendations for treatment of ophthalmia neonatorum were updated in 1982 and widely distributed through state health departments, schools of nursing, and the press as well as by the Centres for Disease Control.

The Society continues its work with industry through the promotion of the Wise Owl Club—a safety incentive programme which is now established world-wide. It has also issued warnings on sports eye injuries and recommendations for eye protection, and expanded its work with industry in reaching not only the employees but their friends and families with a year-round off-the-job eye safety and health programme which includes monthly eye topics and news releases for company publications as well as Society pamphlets and brochures.

One of the Society's most exciting projects for the 1980s is the mass vision screening via the home television set. A broadcast on a national television station in July 1982 was seen by more than 7 million people and has indicated that the TV Eye Test may well become a landmark in health education. As a supplement to mass vision screenings via television, and on the recommendation of a Society Task Force on Adult Vision Problems, the Society has developed a Home Eye Test for Adults. The new test, like the Society's tremendously successful Home Eye Test for Preschool Children, advises arranging a professional eye examination immediately if any section of the test cannot be read properly. More than 9 million copies of the Home Eye Test for Preschool Children have been distributed world-wide and have been reproduced in Spanish, German, Chinese, and Arabic.

The Society's grants for basic and clinical research have fostered significant contributions to the prevention of blindness. This year, the Society doubled the maximum size of its grants from $5000 to $10 000 per year. A Wellcome Research Fellowship, supported by the Burroughs Wellcome Fund, to provide research training for a physician who has completed a residency in ophthalmology, will be administered by the Society beginning in 1983. It will provide a stipend and expenses of $20 000 annually.

The Canadian National Institute for the Blind and the United States

National Society co-operate closely in sharing information, materials, and evaluation of programme results.

North American aid overseas

The United States and Canada, at government level and through non-governmental organizations (NGOs) provide extensive help for prevention of blindness programmes in many developing countries. Information about various of these programmes is given throughout this publication. The NGOs concerned include: Helen Keller International, the International Eye Foundation, Operation Eyesight Universal, and the SEVA Foundation. Brief details of their activities are provided in Supplement B.

SOUTH-EAST ASIA

Dr A. S. M. Lim of Singapore has reported that, while blindness is generally not a major problem in South-East Asian countries, due to the region's relative affluence, pockets of neglected rural communities exist which would benefit from intervention. Overall, it has been estimated that South-East Asia suffers from the almost universal problem of insufficient ophthalmologists. Private practitioners are concentrated in the major towns leaving the rural areas almost devoid of specialist services.

The two most common preventable and curable causes of blindness in South-East Asia are xerophthalmia and cataract. Xerophthalmia is a major cause of childhood blindness in several rural parts of the region, whereas cataract is a condition affecting the majority of South-East Asian countries with the exception of Singapore.

Prevention of blindness activities are promoted within national programmes, which include:

1. Increased efforts made by national organizations to collect information.
2. When priorities have been identified, immediate national action is taken with the co-operation of the World Health Organization Regional Office or non-government organizations.

Several prevention of blindness projects have been carried out in South-East Asia in the past five years. These include:

1. Training and continuing education programmes to improve ophthalmic care at different levels. One of the successful programmes has been the training of 10 Bangladeshi doctors in cataract surgery and general eye care. A 10-week course (conducted by doctors from South-East Asia and Australia) was held in Singapore in 1979. This was followed by field training in Bangladesh. It is satisfying to record that the programme is continuing on an annual basis.

Two successful teaching courses have also been organized, one on 'Recent Advances in Ophthalmology' in 1979 and another through 'The Retina and Laser Photocoagulation Meeting' in 1981. Each was attended by 100 ophthalmologists. The retinal meeting led to the formation of the South-East Asian Fluorescein Angiography Club to deal with retinal diseases. These are becoming an important cause of blindness in South-East Asia as a result of increasing affluence.

Preliminary discussions have started with the Department of Public Health and Social Medicine of the National University of Singapore to establish a Master of Science degree in Public Health Ophthalmology. However, a final decision will depend on the response to similar courses already being held in Baltimore, USA, and London.

Another activity with which the region has been associated is Project Orbis, an American-based international programme. Dr Lim reported that while some workers have reservations regarding this initiative he considered Project Orbis a unique, spectacular, refreshing, and futuristic method of ophthalmic education.

2. A major task within the region is fund raising. To this end, the Asian Foundation for the Prevention of Blindness (AFPB) was formed in February 1981 under the leadership of Mr Karl Stumpf. Based in Hong Kong, the AFPB is responsible for fund raising to support programmes on prevention of blindness.
3. The South-East Asia region has also been responsible for launching an official colour ophthalmic journal for IAPB. The publication of *Vision* has been one of the major projects of IAPB. The journal aims to inform ophthalmologists and other workers of the world's major blinding conditions, which are often well understood but unsatisfactorily controlled.

   The first edition of the publication was well received but as hundreds of copies were distributed free, it proved difficult to maintain its financial viability. Arrangements are being made for a medical publisher to undertake the production. It is intended that once the financial problem is overcome *Vision* will be produced annually.
4. The region is also active in the collection of data concerning ongoing programmes for prevention of blindness.

Indonesia

Indonesia has a total of 1.3 million (1 per cent) blind or visually impaired persons, according to a Department of Social Affairs Census conducted in 1982. Indonesia's major blinding conditions include infection, xerophthalmia, and cataract.

The Government of Indonesia together with the Indonesian

Ophthalmological Association has adopted Primary Eye Care as a part of an integral Public Health Service. A committee for eye health and the prevention of blindness has been set up at village level. This includes the training of auxiliary personnel, primary school teachers, and others.

Helen Keller International together with the Indonesian Government and the Asian Foundation for the Prevention of Blindness has conducted an extensive xerophthalmia programme. The population is being educated on the dangers of vitamin-A deficiency, and has been told how to distinguish the fruits and vegetables in their country which are rich in the vitamin (e.g. mango, papaya, turnip, sweet potato, etc.).

Malaysia

Between 1979 and 1981 mobile clinics of the Malayan Association for the Blind carried out 13 projects. Nearly 30 000 cases were screened in the Operation Cataract campaign and over 290 cases were given operations.

Plans are underway to develop a Home Eye Test for Preschool Children, as well as a $5 million Eye Care Project.

Singapore

The extent and causes of blindness are more comparable with that of developed countries. In 1980 the incidence of blindness in Singapore stood at only 45.8 per 100 000 (0.045 per cent), with 1095 registered blind persons. Similar to the developed countries, the major causes of blindness are congenital and developmental, followed by retinal diseases (myopia, diabetic retinopathy) and glaucoma.

Singapore places priority on the continual upgrading and training of personnel both at the Eye Department and in institutions overseas. An Eye Foundation is envisaged to promote ophthalmic research and subspecialization.

Thailand

It is estimated that there are 200 000 blind persons within a population of 45 million (0.44 per cent), most of whom suffer from cataract. A backlog of cataract is due to the paucity of ophthalmologists.

The World Health Organization sponsored a National Seminar in Bangkok on Restoration of Sight to the Curable Blind. Efforts were made to strengthen eye units at regional, provincial, and district levels. Emphasis has been placed on primary health care, with village health volunteers trained in district hospitals.

The fifth Five Year Plan (1982-6) aims to establish eye clinics in all 72 provinces as compared with the present 37.

In 1979, the Ministry of Health, with the collaboration of Mahidol University, launched a 6-month crash course training programme for surgeons in cataract and emergency glaucoma surgery, increasing the number of ophthalmologists at the provincial and regional hospitals from 22 to 54.

In addition, the establishment of an Institute of Public Health in Ophthalmology is also underway. Its future role may be as a regional centre for prevention of blindness in South-East Asia.

SOUTHERN ASIA

Dr R. Pararajasegaram described the four major developments which highlight prevention of blindness activities in the countries of the region, which now also include Bhutan.

1. A heightened awareness among health policy makers of the vital importance of including and supporting eye care activities in national health planning. This has been made more imperative by the political will and commitment of the elected representatives of the people. For instance, in India prevention of blindness has been included in the government's 20-point programme for socio-economic development.
2. Every country in the region, with the exception of Bhutan, has formulated a National Plan of Action and its implementation is in progress. National committees have been constituted, and national focal points have been identified. The latter not only help co-ordinate activities within the country whether by governmental or non-governmental organizations, but also serve as a linkage with regional and international agencies.
3. An ophthalmologist has been appointed at the WHO Regional Office for South-East Asia in New Delhi with responsibilities for the Regional Prevention of Blindness Programme. This appointment, necessitated by the increased momentum of the programme in the South-East Asia region, was made possible through funding provided by the Royal Commonwealth Society for the Blind and the Asian Foundation for the Prevention of Blindness.
4. As an outcome of a south–south dialogue a South Asian regional committee has been constituted. This regional committee of foreign secretaries is a forum through which the socio-economic aspects of health programmes including eye care are looked at, and the following activities undertaken:
   (a) identifying the constraints found in each country;
   (b) outlining the strategies that can overcome such constraints;
   (c) formulating specific plans based on these strategies; and
   (d) funding these programmes under Technical Cooperation among Developing Countries.

   The prevalence rate of blindness in the region ranges from 0.6 per cent in Sri Lanka to 2 per cent in Bangladesh. These are average figures for the countries—in each country there are underserved areas and impoverished communities where the rates are much higher.

It is estimated that a total population of approximately 853 million in the South Asia region the total number of blind persons is 12 million. In individual countries, the relevant approximate figures are as follows: Bangladesh 1.6 million, Burma 0.5 million, India 9.8 million, The Maldives 1500, Nepal 120 000, and Sri Lanka 90 000. Although data on Bhutan is lacking it is estimated that 25 000 of the country's 1.3 million population have visual impairment. These figures relate to the WHO definitions of blindness, if the number of unilateral blind are taken into account the numbers are even more staggering. In Nepal, for instance, where the most accurate statistics are available, 233 612 people are estimated to be blind in one eye. It is not unlikely that the magnitude of unilateral blindness would be similar in other countries of the region.

In considering causes of blindness, cataract accounts for the largest number of blind people, including those who are unilaterally blind. Cataract is responsible for an average of 65 per cent of the blind population, except in Burma where the figure is relatively less. Of the other causes, infections including trachoma, xerophthalmia, injuries, glaucoma, congenital and hereditary diseases, and posterior segment disorders figures prominently. This group includes a large proportion of the preventable blindness in the region.

Taking cataract as a case in point, it is estimated that in the South Asian region as a whole there is a backlog of about 8 million blind people suffering from this curable condition. To this must be added annually an estimated 1 million new cases. The rapidly increasing life expectancy in the region means that both the annual increase and the number of cataract blind will be likely to more than double by the year 2000. The enormous problem that this curable but unpreventable disease poses, calls for urgent and imperative action, not only in the delivery of presently available technology but also in the development of newer and simpler methods of treatment. More extensive research into the risk factors in cataract—through epidemiological and biochemical studies—may provide clues to its prevention in the not too distant future. If we fail in our endeavours a large percentage of the population, particularly the ageing population, is destined to have their quality of life impaired in their twilight years. Adding 'life to years' will come to have little meaning unless it is possible to also add 'sight to years'.

Bangladesh

A National Plan has been formulated and a representative National Council for the Blind has been constituted with subcommittees assigned responsibilities for specific issues such as curative and preventive activities and rehabilitation.

The Institute of Ophthalmology, Dhaka, not only provides technical leadership and guidance for the national programme but will also assist in the training of various levels of eye health personnel, and encourage both basic and applied research.

Voluntary organizations, chiefly the Bangladesh National Society for the Blind, actively supplement the governmental programme through their branch institutions.

Following the First General Assembly, IAPB formed an 11 member national organizing committee. This now functions in close co-operation with the Ophthalmological Society of Bangladesh and the Bangladesh National Society for the Blind (BNSB). Complementary to BNSB programmes in hospitals, eye camps, and schools, IAPB, as a first initiative has undertaken the training of technical personnel to bring about both a qualitative improvement and quantitative expansion of the programme throughout the whole country. The 37 doctors and 83 paramedics who have so far benefited from such training are working in seven BNSB base eye hospitals and in more than 200 mobile eye camps held every year in the rural areas of Bangladesh.

IAPB has collaborated with BNSB in conducting mass eye camps. Details of those conducted since 1979 are given in Table 4.1.

Table 4.1

Year	Patients treated	Patients operated
1979	137 354	17 415
1980	197 971	26 121
1981	188 006	28 603
1982 (to 30/9)	163 074	25 512

During the last 4 years, the organizing committee of IAPB in Bangladesh received financial assistance from the Agency, the Royal Commonwealth Society for the Blind, and the Australian Government in partnership with the Overseas Prevention of Blindness Committee of the Australian National Council for the Blind as well as technical support in the form of teachers and teaching aids for the programme from Australia, India, Singapore, Sri Lanka, and the United Kingdom.

A building to house the Institute of Public Health Ophthalmology is under construction in Chittagong with the active support of Andheri Hilfe of West Germany. The nutritional blindness programme continues with UNICEF support, while the eye camp programme has received support from the Royal Commonwealth Society for the Blind and Operation Eyesight Universal, Canada.

Bhutan

This sub-Himalayan kingdom, with a population of 1.3 million, became a member of the World Health Organization on 8 March 1982. Although data on the incidence and causes of blindness and visual impairment is not yet available, it is presumed that problems such as blinding malnutrition, infections, cataract, etc., are among the leading causes of avoidable blindness. It is planned to include eye care in the health care delivery system.

Burma

Burma affords an example of the successful implementation of a disease-oriented national programme (for trachoma) prompted by the high prevalence of this blinding disease. The scope of the programme has now been made more comprehensive and, since 1975, has been designated as the Trachoma Control and Prevention of Blindness Project (TCPBP). Burma is also the first country in the region to train and utilize paramedical personnel in eye care activities including lid surgery for correction of trichiasis/entropion. The recent activities in Burma include the strengthening of the eye, ear, nose, and throat hospital at Rangoon to serve as an apex institution for the national programme, and the establishment, with UNDP support, of a regional centre for research into glaucoma, and its early detection at community level. Glaucoma, especially the angle-closure form, has been identified as a leading cause of avoidable blindness in Burma.

India

The inclusion of the National Programme for Control of Blindness in the government's 20-point programme for socio-economic development has provided a major shot in the arm for the programme activities. The government funds for the programme have been doubled. The support of the voluntary sector has been reinforced through more liberal financial assistance and through the streamlining of procedures.

In a review of the national programme, it was observed that in the period 1976-9, there had been a shortfall in services as well as in the establishment and strengthening of the infrastructure. For instance, in 1978, the mobile units failed to achieve the revised downgraded target of 1500 to 2000 cataract operations.

The National Programme for the Control of Blindness in India was the subject of an interim review by a working group in 1981-2. The group identified some of the constraints and bottlenecks in the implementation of the programme, and suggested a mid-course correction particularly in respect of priorities for action. Even prior to the working group's recommendations, a change of priorities instituted in 1979/80, particularly in respect of training of personnel, had contributed to the programme gaining momentum. The goal of the programme is to reduce the prevalence of blindness from the present level of 1.4 per cent to less than 0.5 per cent by the year 2000. To achieve this objective, the following strategies are planned.

1. Manpower development: the training of all categories of eye health personnel will be stepped up to meet the requirements of the programme. For instance, it is estimated that 18 000 eye surgeons will be required by the year 2000 on the modest basis of one for 50 000 population. The present number available is about 5000. Ophthalmic Assistants, who will provide the backbone for the community-oriented eye care services, will number about 2000. Training programmes for achieving this output are now underway in 37 institutions. There will also be a stepping up in the training programmes of all other eye health care personnel.
2. Provision of supplies and equipment: these will include essential drugs for all levels including primary health centres, low-cost spectacles for aphakics, presbyopes, and school children, low vision aids, surgical instruments, and ophthalmic equipment.
3. Institutional infrastructure: emphasis will be laid on primary eye care as an integral part of primary health care (PHC). Concurrent with the strengthening of PHC to meet this need will be the establishment, when necessary, and strengthening of existing District Ophthalmic Services, Mobile Units, Medical Colleges, regional and state Eye Institutes and the Dr Rajendra Prasad Centre for Ophthalmic Sciences. Special emphasis is to be paid to the clearance of the backlog of cataract, the control of corneal blindness due to infection including trachoma and blinding malnutrition, research relevant to the blinding conditions mentioned, and rehabilitation. Health education and eye health promotions will constitute a basic component of the entire programme for the control of blindness. The programme stresses the need for the co-ordination of the many voluntary, individual, and organizational efforts being carried out in the country, both to avoid duplication of effort and to ensure quality of service.

Decentralization of decision making to the state level and the institution of modern management methodologies, including the monitoring or programme implementation and periodic evaluation of achievements, are built into the programme.

The Royal Commonwealth Society for the Blind, which has supported eye-camp activities for several years, launched a project against blinding malnutrition in February 1981. This five-year programme, which aims, in 40 communities in 16 States of India, to protect from blindness some 60 000 children at risk, is the largest programme of its kind in the world. Various international organizations are collaborating to finance different aspects of the programme.

The Maldives

A National Plan has been formulated for a comprehensive community-oriented eye care programme to encompass the whole country. The main initial thrust will be a project to clear the backlog of cataract which is estimated at a thousand cases.

The cataract project for which the World Health Organization will be the executing agency, is being funded through the International Agency for the Prevention of Blindness. A preparatory visit made by the Director of the Aravind Eye Hospital, Madurai, South India, in early September 1982, established the feasibility of the project, and the first batch of about 300 cases of cataract, amongst other conditions, were scheduled to be operated on commencing January 1983 by a surgical team from Aravind Eye Hospital.

Nepal

The Nepal Programme for the Prevention of Blindness, conducted under the auspices of the Government of Nepal and the World Health Organization is described more fully on p. 78. The highlights of the programme are the nation-wide survey which has yielded information not only of the prevalence of blindness (0.84 per cent), its causes, i.e. cataract, infections including trachoma, glaucoma, blinding mulnutrition, etc., but has also provided an in-depth insight into the sociological, environmental, and other risk factors underlying many of these diseases together with their geographical and ethnic distribution. Such information is invaluable in planning interventions for their prevention and control.

The training of different levels of manpower needed for the implementation of the programme activities in a country with an acute dearth of trained personnel has been given top priority. The training has been so tailored as to ensure that the trainees provide a service whilst in training in the field.

Sri Lanka

The National Plan envisages a comprehensive eye care programme as part of the general health care delivery system. Whilst the State provides ophthalmic services through its pecialized institutions and units, voluntary organizations, for example Eye Care Sri Lanka, Sri Lanka Council for the Blind, Assistance to Blind Children etc., supported by agencies such as the Royal Commonwealth Society for the Blind, Operation Eyesight Universal (Canada), Christoffel Blindenmission, and Helen Keller International, increasingly provide outreach services, particularly cataract surgery, and eye health education. A feasibility study on a pilot project for a comprehensive community-oriented eye care service has been carried out by Helen Keller International in collaboration with Sarvodaya. At the time of this report it was anticipated that the project would shortly be underway.

The shortfall in ophthalmic personnel is yet to be made good. Recently instituted national postgraduate training programmes may, to some extent, correct these deficiencies. In the interim period, the Ophthalmic Assistants' Training Institute has plans to commence operation early in 1983. This project has support from the Royal Commonwealth Society for the Blind and the Christoffel Blindenmission.

In conclusion it must be stressed that resources for all these programmes have come from many sources in addition to the national governmental budgets. A number of agencies have supported programmes either through the WHO or through bilateral agreements between governments and local partner organizations. Indeed the donors continual support is vital to the successful implementation of these programmes for the preservation of sight and the restoration of vision.

WESTERN EUROPE

Dr V. Clemmesen presented the report for Western Europe using material collected by Professor G. von Bahr. The magnitude of the problem of blindness in Europe is comparatively modest. The blindness rate for European countries is stated to be between 0.8 and 1.9 per thousand, but it would serve no purpose to quote the figure for each country because the various criteria used are not statistically comparable.

The only country with a high blindness rate is the great arctic island of Greenland. At 3.4 per thousand this is two to three times higher than other European countries. The Eskimo population of about 45 000 is scattered along a 2000 km coast. The most frequent cause of blindness is glaucoma, the area having the highest prevalence in the world of angle-closure glaucoma and senile central retinal degeneration. The prevalence relates directly to the population's high age group which is steadily increasing.

The major causes of blindness in the European region are heredity, diabetes, and glaucoma. In children below 10 years of age, heredity and prenatal or perinatal causes account for 80-90 per cent of blindness. Retrolental fibroplasia, which for a period was a serious cause of blindness in premature babies, has nearly disappeared. Trachoma is almost eradicated, even in southern Europe where only in Greece can a few new cases still be found.

Western European aid overseas

The countries of Western Europe, at government level and through non-governmental organizations, provide extensive help for prevention of blindness programmes in many developing countries. Information about various of these programmes is given throughout this publication. Brief details of the NGOs concerned are given in Supplement B.

WESTERN PACIFIC/OCEANIA

As a result of the expansion of prevention of blindness programmes, IAPB decided to increase its regions from eight to nine. The new region is to be known as Western Pacific/Oceania. At the Second General Assembly, Professor Nakajima was elected chairman of the region. The regional report describing activities undertaken in the countries of the region during the four years leading up to the General Assembly was presented by Professor Billson. Historically, some of the areas now included in this new region had been seen as part of the South-East Asia region. Consequently, Dr Lim, South-East Asia Regional Chairman, has contributed to those reports where there has been a temporary overlap of interests.

Australia

Professor Billson described Australia as a sophisticated country with high technology and professional skills. The government is committed to assisting developing countries in the region, giving high priority to primary health care projects.

Prevention of blindness funding

Funding for prevention of blindness activities in rural Australia is available principally through the Federal Government. The Royal Australian College of Ophthalmologists have been given $1.5 million by the government for an extensive programme in rural eye care. Funding for overseas prevention of blindness comes from two sources:

(a) Bilateral aid sources—the Australian Government has a heavy commitment to overseas aid—the money being given by the Australian Government in response to approach at government to government level. This funding is exemplified in the Bangladesh project where $250 000 was allocated for the eye training complex at Chittagong in 1982. The responsibility for the distribution of these funds has been given to Foresight.
(b) Foresight—The Overseas Aid Subcommittee of the Australian National Council for the Blind (ANCB) has been separately constituted into an organization called Foresight—Australian Overseas

Aid in the Prevention of Blindness Organization. (For further details of Foresight see p. 120.)

Prevention of blindness activities

Rural eye health programme

Phase I 1976-9. The National Trachoma and Eye Health Programme (NTEHP) was developed to conduct a survey of the ocular health of rural Australia, particularly amongst the aborigines. In the course of the survey 100 000 people were examined, more than 1000 operations were performed and 27 000 people were treated with systemic medicine for trachoma. The programme was carried out by the Royal Australian College of Ophthalmologists (RACO), and funded by the Australian Federal Government. Professor Fred Hollows was appointed Director, and more than 80 ophthalmologists donated their time to the programme. An aboriginal man, Mr Gordon Briscoe, who has direct involvement in aboriginal self-help movements, was appointed Assistant Director. One and a half per cent of the aborigines and 0.3 per cent of white Australians in rural areas were found to be blind. In 50 per cent of cases, blindness was due to cataracts and the remaining 50 per cent to corneal diseases in which trachoma was considered to be a prominent factor.

Phase 2. The identification of the cause of blindness in the rural areas enabled strategies for a continuing rural eye health programme to be implemented. RACO is responsible for administering federal funds for the ongoing programmes in the rural areas. State committees have been set up with a majority membership of aborigines and community groups, however, ophthalmologists also participate. Priorities for programmes are determined by each state committee; the programmes are costed and a budget submitted. This mechanism is in keeping with the philosophy of the federal government and the eye profession that responsibility for eye care in the rural sector be determined by the recipients.

Urban prevention of blindness activities

In urban areas the Australian Foundation for the Prevention of Blindness has included screening for glaucoma and visual defects in childhood amongst its activities in different states. In Western Australia, a screening programme for the whole state has been undertaken to survey diabetes and glaucoma.

Prevention of blindness overseas

During 1981 and 1982 doctors from neighbouring countries received work experience in Australia. The doctors came from Thailand, the Philippines, Fiji and Papua New Guinea. The Australian Government is investigating the capacity of the Australian medical profession and universities to be further involved in training doctors from overseas, and is prepared to fund viable proposals, particularly where these would have an impact on primary health care. The government is also supporting proposals for more specialized skills. It is recognized that training diplomas and certificates in the countries where service is to be given are more likely to build national confidence and pride, and to increase the chance that those trained will ultimately practice in their own countries.

Australia is also involved in prevention of blindness programmes in Papua New Guinea, Fiji, the Solomon Islands, and other Pacific islands.

China

China has a population of one billion people, with about 8000 ophthalmologists of the first grade as well as ophthalmologists at second and third grade levels. The leading cause of blindness is cataract, followed by infection and glaucoma. The percentage of blindness is about 0.6 per cent (600 per 100 000). With financial aid and technical expertise from the World Health Organization and social organizations, a prevention of blindness pilot project in Hua Rou county of the Beijing suburb has begun. Should this project prove successful, similar programmes will be initiated to reach even larger segments of the predominantly rural population. The health services are effectively structured with good equipment and financial backing. Prevention of blindness activities are reported to be doing well.

Hong Kong

The number of government registered blind persons stands at 703, of which the majority suffer from cataract, glaucoma, and retinal diseases. The estimated blind population is 0.1 per cent (100 per 100 000). The government leads the fight to prevent blindness, providing a network of eye centres and clinics throughout Hong Kong. There is active participation from local non-profit organizations such as the Hong Kong Eye Bank and Research Foundation which supplies fresh or preserved corneas free. The Peninsula Jaycees also operate a yearly Eye Protection Campaign.

Japan

Eye care services for visually handicapped people in Japan are sophisticated and comprehensive. Despite having a large population only a small area is underserved and the country is not reliant on outside help.

In Japan, funding for overseas prevention of blindness comes from two sources.

1. Bilateral aid sources—this is the principal form of financial support

for overseas prevention of blindness, the money being given by the Japanese Government in response to approaches at government level. This form of funding is exemplified in the Bangladesh project where US$200 000 were allocated for ophthalmic instruments in 1981. Recently, an onchocerciasis project was funded in Guatemala.
2. The Sarahsawa Shipbuilding Foundation—this is a non-governmental organization which has given money to the WHO extra-budgetary fund; a proportion of this gift has been requested to be used for the prevention of blindness activities. Japan is also involved in the training of foreign doctors in ophthalmology, principally from China.

Papua New Guinea

In co-operation with Christoffel Blindenmission (CBM), Helen Keller International (HKI), and the Royal Commonwealth Society for the Blind (RCSB), Foresight in Australia is co-ordinating prevention of blindness activities in PNG, where cataracts and eye injuries are the principal causes of blindness, and where the difficult, mountainous terrain separated by rivers, swamps, and sea are formible barriers to the delivery of services. Foresight is equipping four eye departments that will serve each of the four regions between which the 3 million population of PNG is divided. Notably, it is developing a department at Garoka in the heart of the rural area, with access to 40 per cent of the rural population of PNG. Dr Peter Korimbo, the first national Papua New Guinean to be trained in ophthalmology, having completed two years of training in PNG, went on to undertake a year of work experience with Professor Coster at Flinders University, before returning to take the postgraduate diploma in ophthalmology at Port Moresby University. He will be the first national to gain this diploma and desires to practise in Garoka.

Foresight has paid for two trainers (in visual mobility and rehabilitation) to go to Fiji to assist in training paramedics there with the co-operation of HKI. Two of the people trained under that programme will return to PNG, and one will work in Garoka in association with Dr Korimbo.

Philippines

This is a country of 40 million people with 400 ophthalmologists; 380 of these are in Manila leaving only 20 distributed elsewhere. Prevention of blindness activity is poorly organized for a large rural population which is underserviced and for whom xerophthalmia is a serious burden. Other major blinding conditions are cataract, injuries, glaucoma, and infections.

Solomon Islands

The population of the islands is one million. Since 1968, Dr J. Galbraith, backed by federal government funding, has taken an Australian team to the islands with the principal purpose of performing cataract surgery. The programme has been effective in dealing with the burden of blindness due to cataract, and in recent years has increasingly involved the local population in the delivery of these services, although, because of shortages of local medical personnel, the surgery is still performed entirely by expatriates.

South Korea

In a country with 40 million people, and an estimated number of 100 000 blind people (about 0.25 per cent), the prevalent causes of blindness include cataracts, glaucoma, retinal disorders, and corneal opacities secondary to various accidents. While trachoma and keratomalacia have been almost totally eradicated, there is an increasing proportion of systemic diseases leading to manifest blindness from vascular and diabetic retinopathies, and congenital diseases associated with cataract and glaucoma.

The present available facilities include 500 ophthalmologists with a further 100 in training and 17 medical colleges with ophthalmological departments.

The activities to prevent blindness are mainly carried out by the South Korean Association for the Prevention of Blindness, a voluntary organization inaugurated in 1973 following interest created by the 'Eye Day Movement'. This was conducted by the South Korean Ophthalmological Association for the Prevention of Blindness which is engaged in national programmes, and is also concerned with public education.

Vietnam

With a population of 50 million people Vietnam is regarded as being in need of help in prevention of blindness activities. There are 600 eye doctors but a need exists for 2000; lack of manpower is a serious problem. The USSR has assisted Vietnam in prevention of blindness programmes. Trachoma has been eradicated, and about 70 per cent of Vietnam has been provided with ophthalmic services.

5
Development of national programmes

The concept of a global strategy for the prevention of blindness is being practically expressed through the development of national programmes where the aim is no less than basic eye care for all within a realistic time-scale. Indeed, it is in those countries where national programmes have been established that the most progress in preventing blindness is being achieved.

Sir John Wilson, Honorary President of the International Agency for the Prevention of Blindness, in commenting on the growth of national programmes said 'It is no coincidence that in practically every country where a national programme is now in operation, the preliminary action was taken by a national committee for the prevention of blindness. The fact that such committees, linked to the Agency, now exist in over 50 countries should provide a strong base for growth in the future.' He further urged those members of the Agency attending the Second General Assembly, whose countries did not have an effective national committee, to make the formation or strengthening of such a committee a personal commitment and obligation.

This chapter contains the papers, somewhat condensed, delivered at the Second General Assembly, describing from the authors' personal experiences various aspects of setting up and running national programmes for the prevention of blindness. The papers are followed by relevant recommendations made during the course of the Assembly.

HOW TO DEVELOP A NATIONAL PROGRAMME
M. Mohan

The development of a national programme for the control of blindness is dependent predominantly upon 'three wills'. The political will, the professional will (health planners), and the people's will. Any one of these three wills may be sufficient to generate the necessary interest to provide for the initiation and formulation of a programme. However, co-operation and co-ordination of all three 'wills' is essential for successful implementation of a programme.

Usually it remains for the professionals and health planners to determine how health services can be improved, and to make relevant proposals for the consideration of political and administrative authorities.

In setting out strategies and priorities I will draw on experience and quote examples from the Indian national programme. Formulation of the Indian programme started with a national policy pronouncement by the Central Council of Health at its meeting held in April 1975. It reads as follows: 'One of the basic human rights is the right to see. We have to ensure that no citizen goes blind needlessly, or being blind does not remain so if, by reasonable deployment of skill and resources, his sight can be prevented from deteriorating, or if already lost, can be restored.'

Plan formulation

To formulate a national plan the first steps are to assess the magnitude of the problem and to identify the major causes of blindness (preventable, curable, and incurable). It is also necessary to ascertain regional distributions of the conditions (noting high prevalence), classified by age and sex. The organizational, political, socio-economic, and demographic situation must be taken into account, as well as general health standards. Where no actual committee for the prevention of blindness exists it would be helpful to constitute such a body to plan and co-ordinate all prevention of blindness activities.

Ideally the plan for control of blindness should form a part of a comprehensive health care programme. In India, the problem of blindness was assessed by a sample survey conducted by the Indian Council for Medical Research. The magnitude of the problem was projected in terms of economic loss. The objectives and plan of action were prepared. Various possible constraints and potential obstacles were identified, while, at the same time, existing and potential resources were assessed before the plan was adopted.

The following general guidelines are used for planning a national programme.

1. It is necessary to have at least an estimation of the magnitude of the problem, as well as an assessment of resources including those available from the existing infrastructure, the government, and the various voluntary and private sector organizations involved in health care delivery.
2. The programme should encompass in its activities—planning, strategy building, implementation, monitoring, and feedback from the centre to the periphery and vice versa.
3. The programme should maintain links laterally within the health and concerned non-health sectors.
4. Priorities within the programme should be defined and plans for short-term and long-term goals should be spelt out.
5. The development of manpower and infrastructure facilities should be planned within a time framework, taking into account the stages of the programme leading to total population coverage.
6. All the activities under the national programme should be properly controlled and co-ordinated by appropriate committees and administrative organizations.

The development of a national programme, being a dynamic process, needs to have repeated situational analysis and objective concurrent evaluations undertaken to allow for restructuring and recasting of strategies where necessary.

In the early seventies, with the decline in blinding trachoma in India, it became apparent that more than 50 per cent of blindness was due to an accumulation of people suffering from cataract. Also, with the elimination of smallpox, blindness in children due to keratomalacia became relatively more prominent. This led, in 1975, to the launching of the national programme for the control of blindness, with which the then existing control of trachoma programme was merged.

Health services planning

Health services planning is an integral part of general socio-economic planning. It should be flexible to meet local needs. While there can be a variety of approaches depending upon the prevalent political, economic, and social conditions, it is essential to develop health systems by applying modern planning techniques, for example:

(a) health problem priority index (Q index);[1]
(b) cost benefit analysis; and
(c) performance budgeting.

In deciding the main thrust of the programme, health planners have to decide whether to attempt a comprehensive health care programme or whether they should adopt a more pragmatic approach and concentrate on building strategies for controlling the most pressing problems, by identifying priorities within the programme.

India, it may be noted, adopted a more pragmatic approach following the report of the Health Survey and Development Committee (Bhore Committee) which was appointed in 1946 to assess the health situation. It proposed the institution of national programmes for serious communicable diseases. As a result several national programmes were launched between 1952 and 1955 including those for the control of malaria, smallpox, tuberculosis, cholera, and filaria.

In 1960 blindness was identified by a National Survey and Planning Committee (Mudaliar Committee) as a national health problem, with an estimation of 1.5 blind persons per 1000 population (partial blind not included). The Committee identified trachoma, smallpox, and other eye infections as important causes of blindness. A national trachoma control programme was started in 1963, based on the recommendation of this Committee.

Choice of strategy and alternatives should be planned according to the magnitude and relative weight given to each cause of blindness, the

[1] Q index is used to establish disease priorities. It is calculated by assessing several measurable factors combined in an effort to achieve a quantitative basis for comparing problems. (Michael J. M., Spatafore G. and Williams E. R. (1967) *An Approach to Health Planning*, Public Health Reports, Washington 82, 1063, quoted in *Approaches to National Health Planning* PHP no. 46 WHO.)

extent of technical and other facilities available and possible resources available for mobilization. The Indian programme identified a backlog of cataract, trachoma, and other ocular infections leading to corneal blindness, and nutritional blindness (xerophthalmia) as the priority areas.

In planning strategies, emphasis was laid on community participation and full utilization of voluntary, charitable, and other nongovernmental organizations.

The following strategies were adopted by the Indian National Programme for implementation.

1. The creation of a vertical infrastructure up to the intermediate level and then merging this into the general health services at the periphery.
2. The training of paramedical ophthalmic assistants to provide primary eye care, including refraction of the eye at each primary health centre (PHC), covering about 100 000 people. The training comprised 6 months institutional training and $1\frac{1}{2}$ years of supervised training in a field practice area (mobile unit, district hospital, and PHC).
3. The use of mobile units: services remain inaccessible to people living in remote areas because of problems of communication and lack of transport facilities. The only way to overcome this problem is to use mobile units. However, it must be borne in mind that such a service lacks continuity and poses difficulties in monitoring. Such approaches have been used in immunization and cataract relief programmes in the past. This aspect has been strengthened under the National Programme for the Control of Blindness where a comprehensive eye care approach has been adopted which includes eye health education and treatment of all types of eye diseases by optical, medical and surgical intervention.
4. Providing community-based drugs: another approach which has been very successfully tried in the Indian programme is the community-based distribution of drugs. The antibiotic tubes of ointment used in the trachoma control programme were primarily distributed through peripheral workers and community depot holders.
5. Providing eye health education services to promote ocular health and prevention of blindness activities.

Setting targets

The setting of targets is an essential part of the planning process. It places the programme within time limits and provides goals to be achieved. In the Indian national programme, blindness was required to be reduced from 1.4 per cent in 1975 to 0.3 per cent by the year 2000 with intermediate levels of 1 per cent in 1985 and 0.7 per cent by 1990. There is also a need for setting subsidiary levels regarding population coverage, manpower development, creation of infrastructure facilities, and performance per unit.

Linkages with other services

Linkages need to be established with other health related bodies as follows:

1. Ministry of Education—health education for eye care should be built into school curricula and included in extension education.
2. Ministry of Information and Broadcasting—promotion of health may be undertaken through mass education, audio-visual publicity, and production of commercial documentary films.
3. Industry—to encourage the production of requisite drugs, equipment and glasses, preparation of prosthetics, fortification of food with vitamin A, etc.
4. The agriculture sector—to encourage the production and distribution of vitamin-A-rich foods.
5. The Maternal and Child Health and Family Planning sectors—to ensure vitamin-A distribution to preschool children.
6. The primary health care delivery service—to ensure the inclusion of ophthalmic assistants within the service.
7. Universities, medical colleges, and other training centres.

Resource development

When seeking resources health planners have to compete with a host of other interests for funds. Principally these are from non-health sectors such as defence, energy and power, industry, communications, agriculture, education, etc. Support and co-operation of professional organizations, the public, and the press are essential to ensure that a fair share of resources reach the health sector. The gravity of the situation together with the economic loss incurred to the nation can be powerful persuaders in mobilizing political commitment to determine the extent and sources of funds. For instance, it was estimated in 1975 that blindness cost the Indian nation R10 800 million (approximately US$1200 million) annually in terms of loss of production and a similar amount on maintenance costs.

It is essential that the national programme should develop a long-term perspective for the development of technical and ancillary personnel and the mobilization of private and public sectors. It is worthwhile tapping the resources of international agencies for technical aid and resource development, particularly those which have already been involved in service programmes, like the Royal Commonwealth Society for the Blind, the Christoffel Blindenmission, and, of course, the International Agency for the Prevention of Blindness.

Evaluation and review

All national programmes should be evaluated and reviewed every 5 years to note the achievements, identify shortcomings and constraints, to recommend measures to overcome the identified problems, and to suggest desired changes in the planning and implementation of the programme.

The Indian National Programme for the Control of Blindness was reviewed in April 1982 by a working group constituted by the Government of India and recommendations are being processed.

In conclusion the formulation and development of any national health plan has to be thoughtfully considered. Modern health planning and monitoring procedures should be adopted, and the co-operation of all concerned agencies ensured. Experience of other countries should be taken into account when formulating plans and implementing strategies.

EYE-HEALTH-CARE DELIVERY SYSTEMS
R. H. Meaders

The term eye health care reflects a comprehensive, integrated system to provide promotive, preventive, and therapeutic services to prevent loss of vision from eye disease and injury.

A national eye-health-care delivery system should consist of a continuous system of training, supervision, support, and referral services extending from the level of the most rural villages to the central referral hospital(s). Promotive, preventive, and therapeutic eye health services should be integral components of the general health services provided.

The goal of an eye-health-care delivery system is to reduce the prevalence and incidence of preventable and/or curable visual loss to a level acceptable by the community and the country.

The components of eye health services

Promotive

1. To assist communities to recognize the extent of visual loss present, and its socio-economic impact.
2. To make the population aware that eye disease and visual loss can usually be prevented or cured.
3. To encourage early self-referral to proper care for patients suffering from eye disease, injury or visual loss.
4. To stimulate community desire to take positive action in the prevention of avoidable blindness.

Preventive

1. To assess the nature, extent, and causes of eye disease, blindness, and visual loss at the national and local community level (community diagnosis).
2. To educate the community in those individual and group practices and actions necessary to eliminate or reduce avoidable eye disease and visual loss. The proposed activities must be simple, practical, affordable, and culturally acceptable to the community.
3. To assist the community in planning a programme of intervention in accordance with the wishes, goals, and priorities of the community.
4. To provide appropriate training for a member of the community who will co-ordinate and direct the group effort aimed at reducing or eliminating avoidable vision loss.

Therapeutic

1. To train a member selected by the community in the recognition, simple treatment, or appropriate referral of common eye diseases and injury.
2. To provide 'intermediate level' supervision, support, and referral services by the staff of the responsible health facility. This may include such related disciplines as malaria control workers, leprosy and tuberculosis control teams, teachers, agricultural extension workers, and others.
3. To ensure adequate 'secondary' speciality eye services as a referral source within the larger administrative or geographic regions of the country. In addition to providing an appropriate range of speciality eye care (therapeutic) services, such as secondary level eye health workers also provide training, supervision, and support to the staff of the peripheral health facilities by means of regularly scheduled local clinics and teaching seminars.
4. To provide medical and surgical care as close as possible to where the need is greatest. Rural areas usually contain the vast majority of the population, but only a small fraction of medical personnel and facilities. Patients with eye problems are thus faced with travelling long distances to compete for eye care in crowded central facilities at a relatively exorbitant cost in terms of time and money for the patient and his family.
5. To provide adequate 'tertiary' speciality care at more central locations by properly qualified eye specialists (ophthalmologists). Central referral hospitals provide regular supervision, support, and refresher training for staff at the secondary level facilities by means of regularly scheduled consultation visits.

Training

To assist in the development and utilization of appropriate training aids and curricula to train general and specialized health workers in eye health care.

Advisory

1. To advise the Ministry of Health as to the needs and resources available in the field of eye disease and visual loss.
2. To assist the Ministry of Health in the development, implementation, and ongoing administration of a national blindness prevention and treatment programme integrated into the general health care services.
3. To stimulate involvement by political, business, social, and other leaders in the national programme by the establishment of blindness prevention committees or other non-governmental organizations.

Levels of eye health care

Eye health care consists of four levels; primary, intermediate, secondary, and tertiary.

Primary eye care

Primary eye care refers to practical recognition, simple treatment, and appropriate referral provided by a member of the community who has undergone a short training course. Such a primary health worker is taught to recognize and treat simple infections such as conjunctivitis and foreign bodies, and to recognize and refer all cases with significant eye disease, injury, or visual loss to the nearest static or mobile health facility.

Intermediate eye care

Intermediate eye care is provided by health centres or clinic staff, usually medical auxiliary personnel who have had a practical course in recognition and more advanced treatment of a wide range of eye disorders. They will refer more severe cases to a secondary level facility providing speciality eye care. These personnel provide the ongoing training, supervision, support, and referral for the primary eye care workers.

Secondary eye care

Suitably trained physicians or ophthalmic medical auxiliaries stationed in district or provincial hospitals are expected to conduct routine eye clinics, provide mobile consultation visits to peripheral health facilities, and to provide definitive management for conditions such as trauma, cataract, corneal ulcers, pterygium, intraocular infections, glaucoma, and the complex lid disorders, especially those related to failures arising from treatments for trachoma. In their mobile 'rounds', the consultation clinics are utilized as training opportunities. In addition, the secondary level staff assist local clinic staff in the proper training and supervision of the primary health workers delivering primary eye care. The secondary level staff are also responsible for supervising the preventive activities in their area of responsibility.

Tertiary eye care

Tertiary eye care units are usually established in major urban areas or capitals, and may be associated with a medical school. These centres provide a wide range of sophisticated diagnostic and therapeutic services in addition to providing routine eye care for the immediate urban area. This latter function may detract seriously from the ability of tertiary centres to provide necessary referral services, unless the routine clinics are assigned to less highly trained eye health workers. Ophthalmologists in the tertiary care facilities should be intimately concerned with the supervision and recurrent training of health workers at the secondary and intermediate centres. Close co-operation and communication between all levels of eye health care delivery helps to ensure that the co-ordinated programme makes available diagnosis, treatment, and referral services appropriate to the needs and resources of the country.

In addition to the full range of services of a secondary level centre, the tertiary centre may provide such sophisticated services as corneal transplantation, retinal and vitreous surgery, oculoplastics, and ocular oncology (cancer treatment). In addition, research into the nature and extent of eye disease and blindness should be developed and co-ordinated by the tertiary centres. Once the problems causing visual loss are identified, priorities can be set for applied research and strategic interventions as an integral component of overall health services.

Personnel

In order to ensure that the staffing of various levels of eye-health-care delivery points is appropriate, certain considerations should be kept in mind. While ophthalmic specialists are necessary to provide central consultative services, a national prevention of blindness programme can be co-ordinated, administered, and supervised by someone other than an ophthalmologist. This may be a general physician or a specially trained auxiliary.

The success of a national prevention of blindness programme depends on a continuous chain of training, supervision, support, and referral services, extending in an unbroken fashion from central referral hospitals, through provincial and district hospitals, through the peripheral health facilities, into the most rural villages. The role of the various health care workers is summarized below.

Tertiary level

Ophthalmologists. Ophthalmologists stationed in central referral and provincial hospitals must be oriented toward the appropriate use of either general physicians or specially trained auxiliaries to provide care for most of those people needing eye care, both in the central hospitals and in the more peripheral health units.

In addition to providing speciality consultation, ophthalmologists must teach, supervise courses, delivery, and curriculum development, advise the Ministry of Health as to needs and programme objectives and accomplishments, and provide overall supervision of eye health care workers peripheral to the referral centres.

Support personnel. Non-ophthalmologist eye health workers in the referral hospitals should be given the responsibility of handling routine eye clinics in the same fashion as those in secondary facilities. All too frequently, ophthalmologists in central referral settings spend more than 50 per cent of their time conducting routine eye clinics which should, in fact, be delegated to others. Under supervision, the ophthalmic medical auxiliaries in these central facilities should diagnose, treat, follow up and, when necessary, refer to consultation the majority of patients presenting for care. Well qualified non-ophthalmologist eye health workers should also assist in surgery and provide routine postoperative care of these patients. When rotated to the field, they will be more qualified to arrange for definitive surgery during the ophthalmologist's supervisory training and referral visits to the peripheral facility. Under special circumstances and with proper training and supervision, they may be given authority to perform routine cataract surgery and other procedures.

Secondary level

Physicians or ophthalmic medical auxiliaries (OMAs). Suitably trained physicians and/or well qualified ophthalmic medical auxiliaries can provide speciality eye care in more peripheral health facilities. The work of OMAs should always be supervised by physician eye specialists, with regular refresher training. Secondary level eye specialists are expected to conduct routine eye clinics. Cases beyond their capability are either referred to the tertiary centres or held for the regularly scheduled visits of the supervising ophthalmologist, as appropriate. Patients requiring surgery are operated on either by the visiting ophthalmologist or by the OMA under his supervision, or by the physician eye specialist stationed at the secondary level facility.

Eye specialists (OMAs or physicians) visit the outlying intermediate health facility to conduct regular eye clinics, using the opportunity continually to train and retrain the staff in the recognition, treatment, and appropriate referral of patients with eye disease or injury. In conjunction with the staff of the intermediate facilities, the eye specialists assist in the practical training of village health workers in primary eye care.

Eye specialists also conduct regular in-service training for the staff of the secondary facility in which they are stationed. This will include such other workers and disciplines as maternal and child health teams, immunization teams, specific disease control teams, nutritionists, agriculture extension workers, and others. The health staff serving in the general out-patient clinics should receive regular seminars on the recognition, treatment, and appropriate referral of patients with eye problems.

Support personnel. The eye specialist will usually require assistance in the form of a nursing assistant, eye orderly, or clerk, who will be responsible for keeping records, checking visual acuity, and performing specific treatments under supervision. Stocking and re-ordering of needed supplies is best done by the eye specialist to ensure timely replenishment. In mobile clinics conducted in outlying facilities, the local clinic staff should be involved as much as possible so that the occasion may be used as a teaching practical session as well as a referral clinic. The vehicle driver can also be taught to assist in testing visual acuity and orderly conduct of the clinic.

Intermediate level

Physicians and medical auxiliaries. The physicians, medical assistants, clinical officers, and nurses staffing the intermediate clinics should be given practical training in the recognition, treatment, and appropriate referral of patients presenting for care or referred by the village health workers. Simple, clear visual aids to augment and refresh the training received should be available for constant reference.

Village health workers (VHWs) supervised by the staff should be given a short, practical course in primary eye care with the assistance of the visiting eye specialist. The VHW's basic medications should be routinely checked and resupplied. Problem cases should be examined together on the regular supervisory visits of the clinic staff. It is important that these intermediate level facility staff know and understand the referral network for patients with eye problems beyond their capability to handle.

Primary level

Village health workers (VHWs). The VHW should be given a short, practical course in primary eye care. This course should have two main objectives. The first is to teach the VHW and the villagers what the root causes of eye disease and blindness are in their community. If the community so desires, assistance should be given to tackle these specific problems. The second objective is to train the VHW to recognize and provide a basic treatment for common, simple eye problems and to recognize and refer serious eye problems.

Support personnel. In conjunction with the supervising staff from the responsible health facility and other trainers as appropriate, the entire community should be encouraged to recognize eye problems and to consult the VHW for proper care. It is important to include the traditional medical practitioners in health planning, and where appropriate use them in order to ensure community acceptance and compliance.

Integrated eye health services: a summary

In the foregoing discussion, an attempt has been made to demonstrate a continuum of eye health care. Individual patients first come into contact with the health care system via their village health worker, and then are either treated or referred 'up the chain' of the health care system until they arrive at a level where definitive care can be provided.

In order to provide this definitive care in a timely fashion as close as possible to where the patients live, it is important that suitable training be given to the health workers staffing the most peripheral health facilities, where health workers can provide an 'intermediate' level of capability to handle eye problems and serve to support and supervise the village health workers. Problems beyond the capability of the intermediate level staff are then referred to the secondary level facilities, or held for the 'mobile' clinics conducted by the secondary level eye specialists.

The secondary level eye specialists provide definitive management for a wide range of eye disorders, both in their hospitals and by means of mobile clinics in the outlying facilities mentioned previously. It is important that the eye specialists at the secondary level conduct regular training of general health workers in their geographic or administrative area of responsibility, encouraging them to provide routine eye health care rather than passing along to the eye specialists all patients with eye complaints. In addition, they assist local clinic staff in the appropriate training of primary health workers in primary eye care. If the secondary level eye specialist is an ophthalmic medical auxiliary, he should be properly supervised by a responsible ophthalmologist.

Tertiary level facilities are imperative as a support base for health workers who refer cases which are beyond their capability to handle. As the thrust of training of non-ophthalmologist eye workers is to recognize, treat, or refer patients with eye problems, the referral system must be workable and capable of responding to the needs identified through such a programme. As the root causes of many of the blinding conditions encompass multiple disciplines (agriculture, water supply, sanitation, nutrition, etc.), it is important that eye health care services be integrated into the overall health sector services and co-ordinated with related disciplines.

PERSONNEL TRAINING *M. C. Chirambo*

The use of auxiliary health personnel to expand and accelerate the delivery of health services is a well established fact in Malawi and other developing countries. Among the factors responsible for this are limited economic resources, a paucity of education services and trained manpower, and excessive population growth. Professional personnel are expensive, not only expensive to produce, but also expensive to employ. The alternatives are usually stated in terms of the 'philosophy of the best' which implies that from the very start one provides only for professional quality personnel, starting with small numbers and gradually increasing the flow until a total outreach is achieved. However, experience suggests that attaining a sufficiency of professional personnel is not realistic in present-day Africa.

The diametrically opposed 'philosophy of the most' starts on a basis of total outreach, with personnel trained to an educational standard the country can achieve, given limited economic and educational resources. Over the years, as schooling improves, these standards can be raised until professional competence is achieved.

There is a third way which is not a compromise but an amalgam of both and which solves this quality/quantity dilemma. This third way is based on having a two-tier level of trained personnel where the auxiliary will deliver the quantitative requirements, and the professional the qualitative.

The auxiliary has two roles involving working alongside a professional as an 'assistant' or working in a 'substitute' capacity. In the assistant role, he is always under close supervision, and can be relieved immediately if it becomes apparent that the task in hand is beyond his capacity. In the substitute role, the auxiliary is placed in a situation where supervision is remote, irregular, and sometimes non-existent. It is essential, when training programmes are being devised, that this distinction is borne in mind.

Auxiliaries have a wide range of functions to perform, and a considerable responsibility to discharge. They provide an extensive outreach of services at a cost that the country can afford while, at the same time, saving highly skilled professional personnel from being occupied with routine tasks whilst more serious ills are neglected.

Training

Until 1969, there was no provision for ophthalmic services outside the Central Hospital in Blantyre. In an effort to reduce the high rates of blindness in Malawi, it was decided to expand the ophthalmic services to the remote areas of the country through the training of ophthalmic auxiliaries. These auxiliaries are trained to carry out all the activities concerned with diagnosis and prevention of eye diseases.

Trainees are recruited from among interested medical assistants or clinical officers with at least 2 years experience in the health services of Malawi. The course lasts from 9 months to 1 year and includes theoretical and clinical work. The curriculum includes formal lectures and seminars on ocular anatomy and physiology, diseases of the lid, orbit, conjunctiva, sclera, cornea, lens, uvea, retina, and optic disc as well as refraction and spectacle prescription. The emphasis is mostly on the anterior segment of the eye, the diseases of which constitute the major cause of blindness. The didactic curriculum is accompanied by practical experience in the eye clinic, operating theatres, and wards of the hospital. In addition, students are given field experience in district hospitals and health centres, and participate in the training of primary health workers.

Since 1977, the Medical Auxiliary Training School at Lilongwe, has become the main centre for the training of auxiliary health personnel. The school, which has a capacity for 250 students, is adjacent to Kamuzu Central Hospital which, besides other disciplines, has an eye department with an out-patient clinic, an operating theatre, and a 34-bed ward.

On completion of the course, the auxiliary is expected to diagnose and treat ocular infections, carry out refractions, perform simple surgery on lids and conjunctiva, recognize diseases that require referral, maintain epidemiological records, and provide supervision, support and training for primary health workers and other health-related personnel. Selected graduates of this course undergo further training in intra-ocular surgery, such as cataract extraction, under the supervision of the ophthalmologists in central hospitals. The training is conducted by the ophthalmologist, ward ophthalmic sisters, and clinical officers. After completion of the course, the successful candidates are provided with a complete diagnostic and surgical kit, and posted to district hospitals where small static clinics are set up for them. A few of the ophthalmic auxiliaries are attached to mobile eye units.

Training constraints

There are three government ophthalmologists in Malawi and one at a mission hospital. One government ophthalmologist is stationed at Queen Elizabeth Central Hospital, Blantyre, another at Kamuzu Central Hospital, Lilongwe while the third serves as Director of Medical Services for the Ministry of Health. Each is responsible for providing specialist services as well as conducting training courses in eye health care for the auxiliary and nursing training schools.

The large numbers of patients coming to the eye clinics for diagnosis and treatment, far exceed clinic capacity. Little time is available for the ophthalmologist to participate in the didactic and practical training of auxiliaries. These pressures adversely affect the quantity and quality of training. Similarly, scheduled supervision and refresher training visits by ophthalmologists to ophthalmic auxiliaries posted to district hospitals are seldom accomplished. Since 1969, the hospital eye departments have been able to train only five students at a time due to lack of space and shortage of personnel.

Regional training in the context of technical co-operation between developing countries should be encouraged, especially where the epidemiological patterns and socio-cultural backgrounds are similar. If regional training were to be instituted at the Medical Auxiliary Training School, there would be a need for expansion of classrooms and offices for tutors, acquisition of equipment and supplies, and a mini bus for field-work. At the Kamuzu Central Hospital, the out-patient clinic would need to be extended in order to accommodate more students.

KENYA RURAL BLINDNESS PREVENTION PROJECT R. Whitfield

During the past 20 years, the availability of eye care in rural Kenya has expanded remarkably. From beginning with a single ophthalmic clinical officer on a motorbike in 1962, the present rural ophthalmic programme now provides 10 ophthalmologists and 44 ophthalmic clinical officers, working in 31 rural eye clinics, 14 of which have mobile capabilities. The development of rural preventive and curative services has come about through the concerted efforts of the Kenya Ministry of Health (MOH), the Kenya Society for the Blind (KSB), the Flying Doctor Service, Sight by Wings, and the Kenya Rural Blindness Prevention Project of the International Eye Foundation (IEF). The IEF has been actively engaged in this work for the past ten years.

Together with the MOH and the KSB, the IEF Kenya Project has:

(a) defined the prevalence, distribution, and causes of blindness among rural Kenyans and its relationship to nutritional status;

(b) extended and strengthened the capabilities of the MOH to deliver preventive and therapeutic eye care to the rural areas;
(c) changed the major emphasis in rural eye care from the purely therapeutic, hospital-based approach, to blindness prevention through primary eye care, and educational, promotional, and training activities;
(d) developed promotional and training materials for all levels of health workers, including curricula in primary eye care and blindness prevention for use in the seven rural health training centres, the two central medical training centres, and the many schools of community nursing as well as the teacher training colleges. Educational and promotional material has also been produced for school children and the general public;
(e) assisted in developing a community health care programme in Western Kenya, and initiated a new community-based health care programme in Ithima, north of Mount Kenya, using blindness prevention as an entry point;
(f) organized and implemented seminars on primary eye care and blindness prevention for health workers at all levels, both for those in training, and for those on the job in all districts of six of the seven rural provinces in Kenya. Under the leadership of Dr J. J. Thuku of the Kenya MOH, who is responsible for the development of eye care in the country, and Dr A. M. Awan, Chief Adviser in Ophthalmology to the Ministry of Health, plans for further expansion of the existing programme are now completed.

Critically important to this plan is the graduate programme in ophthalmology at the University Medical School developed under the energetic and highly competent leadership of Dr Volker Klauss. This programme is now training Kenyan ophthalmologists who are assuming leading roles in the supervision and implementation of Kenya's national blindness prevention programme.

Thus, the Kenya Government has recognized the importance of blindness prevention, has developed a national policy for the prevention of blindness, and in a unique example of local and international cooperation with non-governmental organizations, is addressing the following four major components for action in developing a national blindness prevention programme.

1. The extent of the problem has been defined, including the prevalence and causes of blindness and their distribution, thus identifying the worst affected communities and the major causes of preventable blindness.
2. Blindness prevention and primary eye care curricula have been introduced to the training programme for the most peripheral

health workers, including community and health care workers through close co-operation between the blindness prevention programme and the rural development programme of the MOH.
3. Significant strengthening of therapeutic services at the district, provincial, and national levels has been accomplished, including the development of highly effective training programmes for ophthalmic clinical officers and for graduate ophthalmologists.
4. The major causes of blindness identified by country-wide surveys, are being specifically addressed.

Cataract surgery—a priority

Cataract has been shown to be the most important cause of blindness, accounting for 43 per cent of all blindness, and 38 per cent of all visual impairment. With a present population of approximately 16 million, a blindness prevalence of approximately 1 per cent ($< 3/60$), and a prevalence of significant visual loss of 3.7 per cent ($< 6/18$), this means that almost 70 000 Kenyans are blind and another 250 000 are visually impaired from cataract. Furthermore, an estimated 14 000 Kenyans become blind, and another 30 000 become visually impaired from cataract each year.

Dr Paul Steinkuller has estimated that, at the most, only 3500 cataract operations are being performed a year in Kenya. Therefore, although the problem of blindness from cataract is recognized and attempts are being made to effectively address it, the backlog of those needing cataract surgery is increasing at an accelerating rate every year.

There are two major constraints to the solution to this problem. The first is insufficient bed-space for cataract patients, and the second is an insufficient number of cataract surgeons available to do the work. Although the first constraint is being addressed by increasing the numbers of beds in existing peripheral district and subdistrict hospitals and building new facilities, much progress in this area could be made if there were more cataract surgeons available to run static eye clinics and perform cataract surgery at the many existing hospitals where there are, at present, no eye care facilities.

The second major constraint is a serious one, but one which can be addressed effectively within the health training and care facilities now present in Kenya: the training and utilization of ophthalmic clinical officers as cataract surgeons.

The use of paramedical ophthalmic clinical officers to perform cataract extraction

Some years ago Dr Carl Kupfer expressed an interest in our experience in Kenya of training paramedical health workers to perform intraocular surgery, particularly cataract extraction. The performance of cataract extractions by paramedical workers is of immense potential value in countries where cataract is a major cause of blindness and where there is a severe shortage of trained ophthalmologists. However in view of the widely held opinion that only ophthalmologists should be allowed to perform this operation, Dr Kupfer urged me to carry out a prospective study comparing the results of cataract surgery performed by an ophthalmologist to those performed by an ophthalmic clinical officer.

Accordingly, the following simple prospective study was carried out in Central Province. Records were kept on the surgical, immediate postoperative, and late postoperative results of 100 consecutive cataract extractions performed by an ophthalmic clinical officer and 100 similar operations performed by the provincial ophthalmologist. Excluded from the study were any patients found to have preoperative signs of glaucoma, uveitis, complicated cataract, intumescent or morgagnian lens, mental instability or with a history of complications during or after cataract surgery on the fellow eye. The period of the study was from April 1981 to July 1982.

The ophthalmic clinical officer performed all his cataract extractions at Nyeri Provincial General Hospital. The provincial ophthalmologist performed 52 cataract extractions at the Nyeri Hospital and 48 at Murang'a District Hospital.

The procedure used was the same for both operators. Each patient was admitted to the hospital 1 to 3 days before the operation. Routine attention included a daily face and head scrub and a daily application of 1 per cent atropine ointment to the cataractous eye and 1 per cent tetracycline ointment to both eyes. On the day of surgery, the patient was sedated with pethidine and thorazine, and 500 mg of diamox by mouth 2 hours prior to surgery. Pupillary dilatation was achieved using 10 per cent neosynephrine. At surgery the patient's face was prepared with tincture of iodine and surgical spirits. First, a topical anaesthesia was administered using 0.5 per cent proparacaine followed by instillation of argyrol drops. Two per cent procaine or lidocaine was used for facial and retrobulbar block.

The surgeon prepared with a soap and water scrub followed by a rinse using surgical spirits. No surgical gloves were worn. Instruments were boiled for 10 minutes initially, and for 5 minutes between subsequent cases. Sharps were sterilized in surgical spirits.

Using a 'no touch' instrument handling technique, a generous limbal-based conjunctival flap was developed, and the anterior chamber (A/C) was entered using a razor blade. A 7/0 vicryl corneo-scleral (C/S) suture was placed at '12 o'clock' and the incision enlarged with C/S scissors. Following a peripheral iridectomy, the lens was removed with a bell erisiphake, using a tumbling manœuvre. Two to six additional C/S sutures were then placed, and the conjuctiva closed. The A/C was not reformed.

Postoperative care included five days in the hospital with trained ophthalmic personnel in attendance. The dressing was changed after 24 hours and then daily until discharge. Atropine ointment was instilled daily, plus steroid-antibiotic ointment if indicated. The eye was covered at all times with a hard shield. The patient was sent home with a supply of atropine ointment for daily use and a shield for use at night. The first clinic visit was two weeks after discharge, the next at six weeks. Results were obtained as indicated in Table 5.1.

Table 5.1

	Ophthalmic clinical officer	Provincial Ophthalmologist
Number of cataract extractions:	100	100
Operative complications:		
unplanned extracapsular	6	3
vitreous loss	5	3
other	—	—
Immediate postoperative complications (24 hours):		
striate keratopathy	16	6
flat A/C	2	—
hyphema	5	2
iris prolapse	—	—
endophthalmitis	—	—
other	—	—
Late complications (2 and 6 weeks):		
wound leak/flat A/C	—	—
corneal oedema	—	—
uveitis	—	—
secondary membrane needing surgery	1	—
other	—	—

Data is also available from another ophthalmic clinical officer and two provincial ophthalmologists working in Kenya, however, this is retrospective and no postoperative information is available. In the case of the ophthalmic clinical officer and provincial ophthalmologist no. 1, all operations were performed in the surgical theatre of a provincial hospital upon patients who appeared, preoperatively, to be routine and uncomplicated cases of senile cataract. In the case of provincial ophthalmologist no. 2, the figures include all cataract operations performed upon adults during a 4 year period. Included in this group are cataracts secondary to trauma, uveitis, glaucoma, and so on, and include all cataract surgery performed on safari, often under quite difficult conditions. The results are shown in Table 5.2. Data in both tables demonstrate quite conclusively that ophthalmic clinical officers can be excellent ophthalmic surgeons.

Kenya has had more than 15 years of experience utilizing paramedical workers as cataract surgeons. This experience has been a richly

Table 5.2

	Ophthalmic clinical officer	Ophthalmologists No. 1	No. 2
No. of cataract extractions	100	445	829
unplanned extracapsular	4 (4%)	21 (4.7%)	47 (5.7%)
vitreous loss	3 (3%)	13 (2.9%)	42 (5.0%)

rewarding one. The many thousands of Kenyans who have had their sight restored by ophthalmic clinical officers have not received 'second rate' ophthalmic care. The surgical results of ophthalmic clinical officers are as successful as those obtained by Kenyan ophthalmologists and significantly better than the results of ophthalmologists operating in Kenya for short periods of time during brief visits to the country, and who are not familiar with the existing conditions.

For a paramedical worker to perform cataract surgery successfully, he must receive careful on-the-job training in the procedure and in the possible postoperative complications and their management. He must operate frequently, on a regular basis, and be supervised by a competent and concerned ophthalmologist. As Dr Klauss stressed in a recent address to the Association of Surgeons of East Africa, 'for a country with limited resources, the advantages of ophthalmic clinical officers working in the place of ophthalmic surgeons (not merely as assistants to ophthalmic surgeons) are obvious and considerable. More can be trained at less cost and in a shorter period of time; their continued support costs are consideraly less; their surgical results are good; and they are more willing to work in rural areas than are ophthalmologists.'

It is highly unlikely that the plans for Kenya to produce 5 new government ophthalmologists a year for the next 5 years will be accomplished. However, enough new ophthalmologists can be trained to man all of the provincial and the larger district hospitals during the next 5 years. If these ophthalmologists then train and supervise selected ophthalmic clinical officers to perform cataract surgery, great strides can be made towards solving the problem of blindness from cataract in Kenya.

EVALUATION OF BLINDNESS PREVENTION PROGRAMMES *F. Hollows*

Once the goals of a blindness prevention programme are specified, evaluation is quite simply the assessment of the extent to which the blindness prevention programme is achieving its goals while consuming its resources. The formula becomes one of goal accomplishment per unit of resource used.

Goal accomplishment may be measured if the goal of a blindness prevention programme is specified in terms of reducing incidence or prevalence of a form of blindness or a pre-blinding condition; then evaluation or ascertaining the true worth of the programme requires comparison of prevalence or attack rates. Such a comparison requires that like be compared with like. This means that the evaluation be done with the same measurements in the same population as were the original estimates of prevalence rates. The best situation, and this is one that is not often available, is that of a total population study done by observers with measured observer errors, using instruments with measured least counts.

It is wise to avoid synthetic classification such as the MacCallan system for trachoma. It is better to compare basic data such as follicle count, presence or absence of scarring, visual acuity measurements, etc. than to use grades or stages made up of different stages of multiple signs. For all measurements used in evaluation intra- and interobserver error must have been considered.

It is possible to give an account of the work of a blindness prevention programme without seriously evaluating its effects on blindness. Miles travelled, people seen, operations done, health workers employed, populations screened, dispensables used, can all be counted and tallied up. It is possible to describe the establishment of primary, secondary, and tertiary eye care systems and institutions. Further it is possible to enumerate graduates in eye care that a system has produced. It is also possible to list and describe fine items of equipment and specialist facilities that have been acquired, and to mention sophisticated techniques that have become available—but all of these descriptions fall short of evaluation.

The sampling method

Often the ideal, that of comparable total population studies, cannot be done. In that case sampling has to take place. Sampling is beset with difficulties, but most of the problems of sampling have been dealt with by some medical or statistically inclined group before. To ensure that like is being compared with like there are basic rules to employ in an evaluation which involve using sampling methods. Basic components of the samples such as size, age, sex, and social class obviously need to be comparable. The evaluation sample should match the screening sample. The distribution of particular variables in the screening sample decide the composition of the evaluation sample for the same variables. It is best to have a preselected sample, that is a sample selected on the basis of age, domicile, vocation, sex, etc. This avoids a major problem of sampling—that of self-selection. The activities of a blindness prevention programme will have effects that will distort the sample, if self-selection is allowed. For instance, if spectacles are provided by the blindness prevention programme, but this provision was not fully known by the population early in the prevention programme when the evaluation examination was done, then the fact that more people are subsequently attracted by the possibility of getting glasses may distort the sample. The opposite can also occur: some aspect of the initial activities may upset a particular section of the population such as the older men, so that a subsequent sample may be deficient in older men. However, the evaluation examination may need to be done on many persons who self-select, so as not to deter the population and achieve examination of the preselected sample.

Evaluation techniques

The use of a control population enables the evaluation of blindness prevention programmes to be undertaken with some accuracy. In this case, attack rates or prevalence rates can be compared in two populations that are different only in that one has had a blindness prevention programme and one has not: such a situation is often difficult to achieve.

The need for a controlled situation appears to be greatest in those circumstances where the particular procedure employed does not produce immediate self-evident short-term benefits, for example when chemotherapy is the major variable being altered in an anti-trachoma programme.

It is possible under certain circumstances to evaluate blindness prevention activities without any significant epidemiological measurement. For example, a particular unit may be performing cataract extractions. As long as preoperative and postoperative visual acuity is measured and the per operative morbidity and mortality is known, it is possible to evaluate simply on throughput per unit cost for such a system.

An example may be given of cataract camp procedures where many thousands of extractions are done at small cost, and with demonstrable improvement of useful vision, then accounting the cost per vision-improved person is the basic evaluation procedure. Whenever a programme is likely to have difficulties in terms of support from authorities and financial backers or if it has controversial aspects, the provision of high service per unit cost is important. Cost effectiveness will be the major defence of such blindness prevention activities in these circumstances. However, the major defect of such procedural activities is that they do not build a local blindness prevention infrastructure. Neither do they incorporate into the local community a blindness prevention cultural strand. Work of this kind merely arranges for the local community to be a passive recipient for donated aid. The effects of such activities persist as long as the donated services are given, when such donations cease, so does the cost effective procedure.

Involving the community

Political change and structural instability often affect blindness prevention activities. The lack of a cultural element in the blindness prevention programme means dependency on outside systems or government sources. When this occurs the programme founders on political change and international relations. This is the major problem affecting government to government projects. The failure of malaria control is a cogent example of a prevention programme that has not been incorporated into the cultural mainstream of affected communities. A blindness prevention programme must become part of the cultural activities of the people. Culture can be described as those activities taking place between humans that enhance group survival. Blindness prevention should be seen not as a gift from some wealthy donor, or some system imported from an industrially superior donor nation, but rather should be seen as arising from activities being undertaken amongst the people themselves.

All human groups have some form of blindness prevention programme or activity. Mostly these are non-formalized and certainly nothing like a Lions Club 'Save Sight' campaign. The extent to which any group has an excess of avoidable blindness will reflect the extent to which its culture is presently inadequate to deal with its own sight preservation. Where a lost of avoidable blindness exists—there also will exist cultural disorganization, discontinuity, and much decay of the social fabric of the group. Blindness prevention programmes in such circumstances, need to become incorporated into the culture of that group as it reaffirms or rebuilds its social fabric so as to better survive and to survive without avoidable blindness.

In evaluating any blindness prevention programme, it is important to assess the extent to which the programme becomes part of the daily activities of the people. As long as these programmes depend on donations from abroad or from above, they will remain fragile and ephemeral; only when they have been incorporated into the cultural mainstream of society will they persist and be persistently effective.

Some of the actions which need to be undertaken to ensure that the programme becomes part of the peoples' activities may appear to the uninformed observer to be irrelevant to blindness prevention. It is essential that the instigators and executives of the programme be identified with the interests and survival of the client population. To do this requires that key programme personnel should directly identify with the group making obvious a strong and persistent commitment. This will only be achieved by taking part in a wide variety of activities, some of which may be superficially branded as irrelevant.

A blindness prevention programme will be evaluated highly if it follows some simple rules.

1. It should provide an immediate low cost, palpably effective service at all stages of its activities. There should be no programme work that does not provide a direct benefit to the people. When the first survey is being done, sight restoration surgery should be done. All evaluation screenings should be accompanied by a service component. People must never be surveyed or counted without being treated.
2. The major components of the programme must be understood, desired by, and controlled by the client community. A blindness prevention programme that is not owned by the people it serves, will not persist.
3. All non-local programme personnel must demonstrate a sympathetic identification with the client population.
4. The prevention programme must become incorporated into the daily activities of the people it serves.

When resources are allocated to systems that do not fit these criteria, they will not only be wasted, but they will impede the development of effective programmes. Resources allocated to schemes that fit these criteria will show a 'multiplier' effect and they will persist. The simplest test of any blindness prevention programme is what happens when all the foreigners and foreign aid has gone.

PROGRAMME FOR THE PREVENTION AND CONTROL OF BLINDNESS IN NEPAL
R. Pararajasegaram

The report on this national programme, which is being undertaken by the Government of Nepal together with the World Health Organization, was prepared by Dr Nicole Grasset, team leader, and was presented to the Assembly by Dr R. Pararajasegaram.

Nepal, one of the group of least developed countries, with a population of approximately 15 million, is land-locked, having borders with India and China. Although blindness was known to be prevalent in the Kingdom, facilities for eye care prior to the start of the programme in August 1980 were available only through eye camps, three rural eye centres, the Nepal Eye Hospital, a charitable institution in Kathmandu headed by Dr R. P. Pokhrel, and through the eye department of the government Bir Hospital.

In 1978-9, plans for a National Prevention and Control of Blindness Project in Nepal were drawn up, and with the assistance of the Seva Foundation, funds were sought to implement the programme. Representatives of different Ministries of the Government of Nepal approved the plan and, recognizing that blindness was a major public health problem which had to be dealt with rapidly, agreed that high priority would be given to the programme. It was decided that the programme would be incorporated into the Health Sector of the National Development Plans, i.e. the Sixth Plan (1980-5), and eventually would be integrated into the basic health services.

Assistance for the programme through bilateral agreement with the Government of Nepal was obtained from the Centre for Disease Control in Atlanta, USA, the Swiss Red Cross, Christoffel Blindenmission, the French Government, the Gurkha soldiers based in Britain (through the Royal Commonwealth Society for the Blind), Operation Eyesight Universal, Canada, the Japanese Government and the Japan Shipbuilding Industry Foundation had given support prior to the start of the programme in August 1980, for the construction of and equipment for the New Nepal Eye Hospital in Kathmandu as well as for the training of Nepali ophthalmologists.

The Government of Nepal is gradually taking over the running costs of the new eye centres/department which are being established during the five-year period and, by 1984, will have started to create adequate posts under the basic health services for the ophthalmic assistants trained by the project.

In August 1980, priority was given to the conduct of a nation-wide prevalence survey and epidemiological study of blindness in Nepal. Five survey teams travelled from mid-December 1980 to the end of April 1981, by jeep, plane, helicopter, and on foot to more than a hundred villages scattered throughout Nepal, carrying out examinations of 39 887 people. The survey showed that there are an estimated 117 623 blind people in Nepal—that is a prevalence rate of 0.84 per 100 population, in accordance with the definition of 'blindness' used by the WHO. A further 233 612 persons are estimated to have visual acuity of less than 3/60 in one eye (1.66 per 100 population). The prevalence rate appears low, but a comparison with the United States shows that while Nepal has a population less than one-sixteenth of the USA, it nevertheless has the same number of blind people if comparable groups are considered. In addition, to combat the relatively greater problems, Nepal has only 16 ophthalmic surgeons, while the USA has a thousand times as many.

The programme's goal is a 90 per cent reduction of all preventable and curable blindness in Nepal and national self-sufficiency in eye care by 1986-7. The programme comprises the following main features:

(a) strengthening of the infrastructure for the delivery of eye care;
(b) training in eye care of personnel in different categories and levels;
(c) establishing in 1986, an eye centre in each of the zones, with secondary centres in some areas;
(d) posting in each zonal centre, at least one ophthalmologist, two ophthalmic assistants, and two trained nurses. Plans have been

drawn up to have a total of 24 Nepali ophthalmologists available by 1986; and
(e) posting one ophthalmic assistant in each of the 75 district hospitals. At least one of the two district medical officers at this level will receive one or more refresher courses in eye care (training course of two weeks). At the peripheral levels, i.e. at health posts (of which there are on average seven per district), and at the village level (approximately 33 000 villages/wards), efforts will be made to train one health auxiliary worker per health post and one voluntary village health worker (called community health leaders in Nepal), per village in primary eye care.

Main practical successes

Training of ophthalmic assistants (OAs) and OA mobile teams

Until late 1981, this category of personnel was non-existent in Nepal. It is planned that by 1986, the country will have a minimum of 94 OAs. They will be posted at:

(a) the district hospitals (one per district);
(b) the zonal eye centres (two per centre); and
(c) the Nepal Eye/Bir Hospital in Kathmandu (eight).

Thirty-four OAs have already received 1 year on-the-job training following an initial $2\frac{1}{2}$ month theoretical training in Kathmandu. Ten more were trained for 1 year at the Aravind Eye Hospital, Madurai, India. The on-the-job training of the OAs was carried out in the out-patients departments and operating theatres of the eye centres, in eye camps, and in mobile units. In addition, 28 OAs were trained in groups for the surgery of trichiasis/entropion (T/E). These 28 OAs made up the four mobile teams which functioned from November 1981 to May 1982 in two trachoma hyperendemic districts in the far west of Nepal. The OA teams, initially accompanied and trained by an ophthalmologist, carried out a house-to-house search for persons either blind or suffering from a blinding condition. Once each of the nine villages/wards making up a panchayat had been visited (one OA searcher per village), on the spot operations, under canvas, were carried out on T/E cases detected. At the same time, and by rotation, two or three OAs were being trained in the surgery of T/E, sterilization of instruments, administration of anaesthetic, etc. Patients were told to come back approximately 10 days later at a determined location to have their stitches out. Absorbable sutures are now being used which have the advantage of not obliging the patient to come back for the removal of stitches. The most skilled OAs, after approximately two months training, began operating on their own, periodically supervised by one of the four ophthalmologists on the spot.

Apart from the detection of T/E cases, the searchers recorded other main blinding conditions encountered and referred these as necessary. They also gave treatment and took preventive measures for trachoma and xerophthalmia, providing first aid eye treatment on an *ad hoc* basis.

Establishment of low-cost centres

Since October 1981, five new eye centres have been initiated or established. Priority was given to the establishment of eye centres in the trachoma endemic west and far western regions of the country where, until now, with the exception of eye camps, no eye care was available for a population of approximately six million.

The Dhangadi Eye Hospital has been entirely constructed by the project with local community participation and support. It comprises two operating theatres, with appropriate adjoining rooms, an outpatient department with four offices and a big waiting room, as well as a ward for 28 patients. The total cost involved is approximately $30 000, using local builders and materials. In addition, two more wards are to be constructed as well as quarters for the staff. In the meantime, because over 1000 cataract patients requiring surgery have been detected in Kailali district alone, it will be necessary to use temporary tented accommodation until the two other wards are constructed.

Apart from catering for the patients coming to the out-patients department, and those having operations, the centre also serves as a base for the mobile units in the terai, for the field clinics being established in five hilly districts, for the training of OAs and basic health staff of the region, and for health education at village level. Four similar low-cost eye centres in other zones are to be established in 1983 on the same basis.

Elimination of cataract backlog

There are presently an estimated 78 605 cataract blind patients requiring surgery and if the estimated backlog of 300 000 to 350 000 cataracts which will accumulate between 1982 and 1986 is, as planned, to be eliminated by the end of 1986, over 60 000 cataracts will have to be operated on yearly, as compared with the few thousand operated on annually in past years.

Since only 16 Nepali ophthalmic surgeons will be available from 1982 until the end of 1985 (eight more will be following a three-year specialization course in India until 1985), it is planned that specialized manpower from different sources will be used during the five-year period, viz:

1. A certain number of district medical officers will undergo three to six months training in cataract surgery.

2. Nepali surgeons will be assisted by an appropriate number of expatriate surgeons working on a totally voluntary basis.
3. Experienced 'ophthalmic teams' from the region (India and Pakistan), will hold eye camps/field clinics, bringing with them all the staff, equipment, and support necessary. These will be recruited on a contract basis.

As the larger proportion of cataract patients lives in the terai plain, where the eye centres are located, these centres will be strengthened; the number of beds will be increased from four to approximately 100 per centre by the use of local buildings and tents or the construction of low-cost wards.

Small secondary eye centres attached to district hospitals which are accessible by plane will begin to be established in the far western region. In each of these, one OA will be posted and an ophthalmologist will fly to the centre at regular intervals, operating for a few days on cataract cases previously detected in the district and referred to the centre by the OA. He will also be able to check, when necessary, the aphakics operated on during his previous visits.

Conclusion

The vast majority of the population is illiterate; there are, furthermore, 71 different ethnic groups, with their specific mores, speaking 52 different languages. As a result, there are difficulties in the training of staff, and in providing health education in eye care for the population. There are also problems of communication between health staff and villagers.

Last, but not least, the non-availability of required funds on a continuing basis handicaps the continuity of the implementation of the programme and the planning of both short- and long-term activities.

THE PRIMARY EYE CARE PROGRAMME IN THE EASTERN REGION OF PERU *Francisco Contreras*

Peru has a population of 18 million, including about 270 000 blind people. The Andean Range, which lies in one long continuous chain from north to south separates the country, geographically, into the coastal area where ophthalmological services are easily provided, the Sierra, Andean or mountainous region, and the eastern region or jungle. The two latter regions in general, having poor inland communications and limited resources for health care.

The aim of the primary eye care programme is to integrate eye care into all levels of the National Health System for the benefit of urban and rural communities, making use of official sectors such as education, communication, labour, etc., and non-official sectors such as the Comision Nacional de Prevencion de Ceguera.

First phase of the programme—Department of San Martin

The programme was initiated in 1978, in the north-east regional jungle villages where ophthalmological care was not provided, and where there is a high incidence of ocular morbidity.

In 1979, 30 primary health workers (auxiliary personnel of the Ministry of Health) were trained in groups of six for 12-week periods. Their objective was to treat the most simple ocular disorders and to promote activities for the prevention of blindness.

Secondary care was provided by a general physician, fully equipped and trained over a two-year period. Unfortunately, this doctor emigrated to Lima, leaving the scheme incomplete. Subsequently, second level assistance was given by resident hospital physicians from the Centro Oftamologico Luciano Barrere, of the Hospital Santo Toribio de Mogrovejo in Lima, under the auspices of the Ministry of Health, which also provides services at the tertiary level.

Second phase of the programme—Department of Puno

In 1980, the Department of Puno (Andean region), where there is a population of one million inhabitants without ophthalmological assistance, was chosen for the second phase of the programme. Twenty-five health auxiliaries were selected under the following criteria:

(a) those already working as health auxiliaries in the community;
(b) those having an elementary school level of education;
(c) those having leadership qualities; and
(d) those having a commitment to work for 2 years in their own rural area.

The health officers of the Department of Puno carried out the personnel selection, and there followed an 8-week training period at the Centro Oftamologico Luciano Barrere. The teaching consisted of eight working units:

(a) geopolitical map and social description organization schedule; description of observed ocular disease; entrance test;
(b) basic ocular knowledge;
(c) learning about eye examination and evaluation of visual function, visual acuity, visual fields to confrontation, eye alignment, eye movement, ocular pressure;
(d) red eye and ocular emergencies; first aid;
(e) activities on prevention of blindness and promotion of eye health;
(f) activities for recovery—what to do and where to refer to?;
(g) activities for rehabilitation; visits to centres of rehabilitation; and
(h) the way to prepare reports.

The teaching included activities in the out-patient clinic, in the ocular pathology laboratory, surgery room, and in hospital wards.

Seven nurses also received 15 days training in developing primary eye care assistance and field supervision.

Four months after completing the training of the 25 health auxiliaries, who were distributed throughout the region, an examination of their work was carried out in the capital city of the region, Puno. In this way the first statistical data was obtained. Though not absolutely precise it was nevertheless significant. As a result the following were reported to be among the major causes of ocular disorders:

(a) accidents;
(b) infectious conjunctivitis;
(c) chronic conjunctivitis (also by snow); and
(d) hordeolum.

It was also noted that ongoing supervision and adequate audio-visual material was needed in order to carry out short refresher courses. The second level for this region will be achieved in 1983 when the training of a local physician is completed. He is currently undertaking a 3-year training programme at the Centro Oftalmologico Luciano Barrere. Meanwhile this level is covered with periodic visits from physicians of the third level.

The appropriate number of auxiliary personnel, nurses, and physicians necessary for the first and second levels will be decided as soon as epidemiology data, already being compiled, becomes available. Other specific actions also await these results.

In April 1982 activities in the central regions (Pasco, Huanuco, and Ucayali) were initiated by training another 25 health auxiliaries and nine nurses. Other initiatives include:

1. The preparation of an official Manual for Primary Eye Care to outline the activities that the health auxiliaries carry out.
2. The preparation of a teaching set (slides, cassettes, working guides) to train personnel at the three levels.
3. Training elementary school teachers of the Ministry of Education in the visual screening and basic knowledge for prevention of blindness, not only in Lima but also in other locations where the prevention of blindness programme is being developed.

In conclusion, in Peru, the development of activities for primary eye care has aroused the interest of other specialities. It is hoped that uniting in a common purpose may benefit the overall health of the community.

In addition, it needs to be said that these prevention of blindness activities would not have been possible without the valued support given by Operation Eyesight Universal of Canada, the Agencia Internacional para Prevencion de Ceguera (IAPB), the Ministry of Health of Peru, and the World Health Organization. Helen Keller International is now also offering economic support.

PRACTICAL PROBLEMS AND SUCCESSES OF THE RCSB CATARACT SURGERY PROGRAMME IN INDIA Rajendra T. Vyas

Cataract is responsible for 55 per cent of the total cases of blindness in India. Furthermore, the Indian Council of Medical Research, based on a survey conducted in 1972-3 by its statistics department, has projected some staggering figures for cataract blindness (vision less than 6/60 with correction), for the immediate years ahead. As Table 5.3 below shows, in 1991 the figure for blindness in right or left eyes is expected to rise to over 24 million.

Table 5.3

Year	Right eye	Left eye	Total
1981	8 892 456	9 126 593	18 019 049
1986	10 405 627	10 680 759	21 086 396
1991	12 248 833	12 583 177	24 832 010

Services, though developing rapidly, remain inadequate and though a remarkable effort has been made to achieve 735 000 cataract operations a year a formidable backlog is accumulating. There are only about 12 000 ophthalmic beds and 4500 ophthalmic surgeons, who work mainly in cities and towns, to cater for an estimated Indian population of 700 million of which 560 million live in rural areas.

Eye camps

Such limited services essentially have to be augmented by eye camps which are able to reach far-flung rural and urban target populations. In this way it is possible to serve areas where a permanent ophthalmic infrastructure is non-existent.

In organizing an eye camp there are a number of practical problems which need to be taken into consideration.

1. Generally eye camps can only be organized in most parts of India between November and March, thus placing considerable strain on manpower resources.
2. Only a limited number of charitable eye hospitals and organizations are willing and able to arrange eye camps.
3. Eye-camp surgery requires special skill and a ready adaptability to working in difficult conditions.
4. There are not enough medical and paramedical personnel possessing the required temperament to work in rural conditions and in situations different from those in urban hospitals.

Despite all these problems, the Royal Commonwealth Society for the Blind (RCSB) launched a campaign in 1970 to help combat the rising numbers of cataracts, and in the following 11 years sponsored eye camps where the eyes of about 8 million people were examined and treated, and where sight was restored to more than 1 million previously blind people. In 1981 alone the RCSB sponsored 2011 eye camps in which 1 095 416 eye patients were examined and treated, and 133 464 cataract operations were performed.

The success rate in eye camps is 90 to 95 per cent, and this is due in no small part to the use of antibiotics, sutures, and modern appliances such as cryo units.

Eye camps also owe a significant measure of their success to service organizations such as Lions Clubs (of which there are more than 200) and Rotary Clubs (over 300), in addition to specially created eye-camp committees.

In the final analysis, the efficiency of eye camps depends on the effective use of eye-camp teams. This can only be ensured by preparing detailed, carefully planned schedules and by a careful selection of locations. In addition, it has been found that organizations having their own ophthalmic surgeons, vehicles, and equipment have a higher rate of productivity.

Eye camps are necessarily transitional in nature. They are to be eventually replaced by 20 to 40 bedded rural-based eye hospitals with an outreach arm of mobile ophthalmic units.

In the meantime, certain steps need to be taken to increase the numbers of patients treated including:

1. The augmentation of the number of eye camps by selecting suitable permanent sites in rural areas throughout the year, instead of the five months currently achieved in most parts of India. Potentially this will double the number of patients undergoing surgery.
2. An increase in the number of ophthalmic beds available at primary health centres and district hospitals.
3. An increase in training programmes for paramedical ophthalmic staff, thus leaving the ophthalmic surgeons more time to perform surgery.

THE CONTROL OF XEROPHTHALMIA IN INDONESIA *I. Tarwotjo and Robert Tilden*

Indonesia, with a population of 150 million people, has made the control of xerophthalmia a major goal within the public health sector. The Ministry of Health recognizes vitamin-A deficiency as Indonesia's largest nutritional problem. Although the country has potentially adequate sources of carotene and vitamin A, many cases of xerophthalmia are still found among young children at health clinics—just as they were reported to have occurred by Professor Ommen in the early 1950s.

Night blindness and Bitot spots, the most common manifestation of vitamin-A deficiency, are well known among the people of Indonesia, particularly those living in the most densely populated island of Java. These ocular signs have been given popular local names, and are commonly known to be associated with heavy worm infestation. A large number of studies have confirmed the high relationship between these eye signs and low serum vitamin-A levels.

A concerted effort to combat this deficiency disease was initiated in the 1960s, by distribution of crude red palm oil to families in a number of rural villages known to be at high risk of xerophthalmia. However, it was found that this method of xerophthalmia control was ineffective, impractical, and unacceptable to the participants. In 1971, after the Hyderabad nutritional meeting, nutritionists in Indonesia became aware of vitamin-A concentrate and a field test was held. Two different doses were tried, one of 200 000 IU twice a year, and the other of 300 000 IU once a year. The 200 000 IU regime was found to be more acceptable. The implementation of this intervention programme was based mainly on clinic and hospital reports, but the true magnitude and distribution of the xerophthalmia problem in Indonesia was unknown until a nation-wide survey was conducted in 1977-9.

From that survey, and from an associated epidemiological study which was conducted in the same period, it was calculated that xerophthalmia was indeed a public health problem of major importance in Indonesia, as well as being the major cause of blindness in preschool age children. Fifteen provinces of the 24 provinces included in the survey were found to be at high risk of xerophthalmia (the population in a province ranges from 5 to 25 million people).

Green leafy vegetables are available for almost all families. It was found in the 1977-9 prevalence study that almost all families of children with xerophthalmia consumed vegetables, even if the children did not. In June 1979, a large feasibility study was held in Jakarta to determine which of all the potentially fortifiable food stuffs was most appropriate for enrichment with vitamin A. The general consensus of the meeting was that monosodium glutamate was the most appropriate vehicle.

Information collected has been useful not only in designing effective xerophthalmia prevention programmes, but also in shaping the third five-year National Development Plan which includes specific health and nutrition programmes as well as the formulation of a national strategy for attaining health for all by the year 2000. In the development plan, the target of the xerophthalmia control programme is to cover 11 million preschool children with the massive dose (200 000 IU) vitamin-A distribution, food fortification, and nutrition education activities.

By the year 2000 the Government of Indonesia hopes to have been successful in reducing the prevalence of xerophthalmia by at least 70 per cent, so that in most provinces nutritional blindness will cease to be a serious health problem.

Current activities to control xerophthalmia

In 1982, the massive dose vitamin-A-capsule distribution was targeted to cover about 8 million preschool age rural children in high risk areas. Distribution was arranged through:

(a) a general nutrition programme presented as an integrated package to be delivered by the health department, family planning or womens' groups;
(b) special capsule delivery systems in villages of high risk areas which are not covered by general nutrition programmes; and
(c) the primary medical centres (Puskesmes) for each district of Indonesia.

In addition, vitamin-A-enriched monosodium glutamate is to be distributed through commercial channels in a pilot area of West Java. Vitamin-A-enriched salt has also been produced and distributed to plantation workers in certain areas.

The topic of the prevention of xerophthalmia is one of the main themes in training sessions for various levels of medical personnel. Nutrition education modules are being developed, implemented, and evaluated in different high risk regional areas of Indonesia. This includes not only attempting to change the behaviour of mothers, but also of schoolchildren and pre-school children.

Special training has been conducted for medical and paramedical personnel of 50 Puskesmes in high risk areas. These sessions were designed to increase the capability of the Puskesmes staff in the detection, recording, and reporting, as well as management of the vitamin-A-intervention programmes.

An objective evaluation of the xerophthalmia control programme is being conducted to determine the coverage of vitamin-A-capsule distribution through different channels, and the impact of the programme. The clinical information from the evaluation study will be used to improve future planning of vitamin-A-deficiency intervention activities.

The role of Helen Keller International in xerophthalmia control in Indonesia

Helen Keller International (HKI) has been working with the Indonesian Ministry of Health for over 10 years on programmes for the prevention of nutritional blindness. We have already described the progress made during this time towards mass prophylaxis, from the distribution of red palm oil to preschoolchildren to the introduction of high dose vitamin A.

It was at this point that HKI, under the direction of Dr Susan Pettiss, assisted with evaluation by providing financial and technical support. The study demonstrated that the 200 000 IU megadose vitamin-A capsule was effective in preventing conjunctival xerophthalmia, but that the programme had support and supervisory problems. The results of this study were presented at a joint USAID/WHO meeting on xerophthalmia held in Jakarta in 1974. In attendance at this meeting was an ophthalmologist who was very anxious to do further characterization of xerophthalmia. In discussions with Tarwotjo and others, a plan of action was developed. In 1976, Dr Alfred Sommer arrived with his family in Indonesia to set up one of the largest comprehensive studies in xerophthalmia ever undertaken. Four basic studies were performed:

(a) a longitudinal study following 5000 children over 18 months;
(b) a clinical study of Bitot spots at Rumah Sakit Mata Cicendo;
(c) a clinical study on corneal xerophthalmia at Cicendo; and
(d) a national prevalence study covering 24 of the 27 provinces.

The significance and output of these four studies are numerous and varied. Apart from the many peer-reviewed articles and the classic text on xerophthalmia, a wealth of data has been generated which has been used for planning effective nutritional blindness control programmes.

In 1977-8 HKI extended its work into the area of integrated education. This programme's goal was to educate primary school age visually handicapped children with their sighted peers.

HKI's goal over the next few years in Indonesia is to consolidate its services to blind people while maintaining its overall commitments to xerophthalmia control, integrated education, and rural rehabilitation services. It aims to explore new ways to promote eye health care, and to continue to work in collaboration with the Ministry of Health while, at the same time collecting information on cost coverage and impact, so that further strategic planning activities can generate a plan of action to eliminate xerophthalmia at minimum cost.

TRAINING AND ROLE OF PRIMARY EYE-CARE TECHNICIANS IN GUATEMALA *Gloria Tujab*

In preventing blindness in Guatemala, as in many developing countries, priority should be given to primary eye-care programmes, in order to cover rural areas that are in need of this type of assistance.

To accomplish this important task, the National Committee for the

Blind has established two specific areas of training: primary eye-care technicians and front-line workers in primary eye care.

Training programmes

The training programme for primary eye-care technicians aims to equip workers to:

(a) detect eye problems, dealing with those for which their training qualifies them, and making any necessary referrals to secondary and tertiary levels;
(b) promote eye health in the communities, employing acknowledged precepts in basic therapeutics, prevention education, and creating awareness in the community, adapted to the Guatemalan environment;
(c) participate in the motivation, orientation and education of persons from the community itself, thereby generating a multiplying effect.

In this role, the primary eye-care technician spearheads action at community level for the elimination of avoidable blindness.

Primary eye-care technicians are selected from among nurses, public health technicians, social workers, midwives, community leaders, teachers, and others. Candidates must demonstrate an awareness of the importance of eye health; a commitment to primary eye care; a willingness to adapt to any working environment; and a strong determination to implement their tasks.

The training period is of three months' duration and uses methods, resources, and techniques most suitable to the environment where the students will be working full-time.

The course consists of theory and practice concerned with the following subjects:

(a) primary eye health care	40%
(b) nutrition	30%
(c) maternal and child care	10%
(d) community promotion	10%
(e) planning and administration	10%

The training of eye care technicians has a multiplying effect when they impart elements of their training to front-line workers in primary eye care. In 1981, 1500 nurses, public health technicians, social workers, midwives, community leaders, teachers, and others were trained in three-day mini-courses. These front-line workers are prepared to contribute part of their time to the maintenance of eye health in their communities. Their effectiveness has been one of the greatest contributions to the success of the programme for the prevention of blindness in Guatemala.

Both primary eye-care technicians and front-line workers, are instructed to make referrals to ophthalmologists for specialized ocular treatment, and are supervised and evaluated periodically by ophthalmologists and other specialized professional personnel.

Delivery of care

Primary eye-care technicians deliver primary eye care to the rural population and to marginal urban dwellers. They travel to remote areas by whatever mode of transport is available—on foot, on horseback, car, jeep or boat. In such areas the communications skills embodied in the technicians training programme is recognized as being specially valuable. Understanding gained in this way can breach cultural differences and gain the trust and co-operation of the people in need of help. Because the population is mostly of Indian origin, sometimes speaking Spanish but communicating more fluently in their ancestral languages, primary eye-care technicians include in their numbers speakers of such major languages as Cackchiquel, Kekchí, Mam, and Quiché.

As a result of previous surveys of the community, the primary eye-care technicians are already aware of many of the relevant characteristics of the community including information on geographic factors, the population's density and ethnic composition, means of communication, socio-economic and religious patterns, educational facilities, sanitary conditions and, principally, any known factors relating to eye health.

On arrival, the technicians seek to motivate the community into an awareness of the importance of eye health and how to achieve it. With the co-operation of community leaders, they give informal lectures on such matters as eye health, nutrition, child care, and sanitation.

Detection of eye problems

The following routine is used for the detection of eye problems:

(a) history of eye problems;
(b) testing for visual acuity;
(c) external examination of the eye with flashlight and magnifying glass;
(d) diagnosis of anterior segment problems;
(e) primary treatment as necessary; and
(f) referrals to secondary and tertiary levels.

Primary eye-care technicians are also trained to help those who are found to have irreversible blindness, by pointing out that visual deficiencies can be compensated for. They carry a slide presentation showing the progress of visually handicapped children who develop their full potential through the National Committee for the Blind's early stimulation programme and specialized education at the school for blind children. They also show the success achieved by blind adults after rehabilitation in the Committee's urban or rural centres; in addition, they show that elderly blind people can be integrated happily into their families and communities through appropriate methods of rehabilitation.

The outstanding devotion of the primary eye-care technicians of the National Committee for the Blind could serve as a beacon to other countries which, like Guatemala, need the services of primary eye-care personnel, to stamp out avoidable blindness

SURVEY AND TREATMENT OF THE BLIND IN ZHONG-SHAN COUNTY, GUANG-DONG, CHINA
Mao Wen-shu, Chen Yao-Zhen, and Guan Zheng-shi

In the spring of 1982, a survey of the blind was conducted in Zhong-Shan county of Guang-Dong Province in the southern part of China. The county contains 25 communes and a town. Each commune has a hospital and there is a county hospital in the town. The total population of the county is slightly over one million (1 009 275).

In the survey, each commune hospital contributed one doctor for one week's training held in the county hospital. They gave lectures on diagnosis and treatment of common eye diseases such as trachoma, cataract, glaucoma, eye injury, etc.

After this session, the local doctors returned to their own communes to conduct concentrated training classes for two days to 372 'barefoot doctors'. The great advantage was that most of these youngsters came from nearby districts where they were familiar with the majority of their neighbours. They were taught to fill in the forms issued by WHO, which were finally carefully checked by the senior eye doctors or the Eye Hospital ophthalmologists. Simple eye clinics and operating rooms were set up in the commune hospital. Those who were curably blind were either operated on or treated medically.

In all, 2407 cases of blindness were found, of these, 1219 were binocular and 1188 were monocular. The ratio of female to male was 1.7:1.0.

Overall, cataract was found to be the leading cause of blindness, but causation varied in different age groups. The most common eye diseases under the age of 25 were corneal leukoma, staphyloma and phthisis bulbi secondary as well as various infectious diseases, trachoma, and malnutrition. The most common cause of blindness in people over 25 years old was cataract, followed by corneal diseases and glaucoma.

Subsequently, 313 major and minor operations were performed— all without complications. Only 54 of these (65 eyes) were for cataract. Unfortunately, the operations were carried out during spring, the busy farming season in Guang-Dong province. Undoubtedly, this was an inappropriate time and explains the low numbers of patients attending for sight-restoring operations.

The survey showed, from the records of each commune clinic, that the prevalence of the common eye diseases differed from area to area. For instance, in Huangpu commune, we observed some severe cases of trachoma, and pterygium was also common. The farmers there subsist in an impoverished state. The people have no electricity or clean water, are short of fuel, and even lack decent clothing. In Xialan, however, where living standards are nearer to that of a small city, and where the social and environmental conditions are good, a different picture was presented. The incidence of ocular ailment was closer to that seen in a city. Throughout Zhong-Shan county, we found the visual loss was between 110 and 443 per 1 million people. Of the total 3626 blind, 1960 were found to be curable. Since the survey was undertaken, services have continued to be provided to treat those people who are needlessly blind or who are at risk of blindness.

RECOMMENDATIONS

Participants at the Assembly of the IAPB agreed the following recommendations for action within national prevention of blindness programmes:

1. The elimination of avoidable blindness being a widely recognized health priority, the IAPB should encourage every country to examine the prevalence of blindness and its eye services.
2. Every country should be encouraged to set goals for the reduction of blindness, and to devise and implement appropriate programmes to achieve these goals.
3. In many countries there is a large disparity between the needs for basic eye care and the number of ophthalmologists that the country has, or can support. Other things being equal, this means that areas that are presently neglected will continue to remain in dire need of eye care including surgery for lid deformities, pterygium, and cataract, unless new approaches are developed.

    The IAPB, therefore, applauds innovative approaches to prevention of blindness programmes and endorses the application of any or all of them in any country in which they are found to be appropriate to the need.
4. Each country with a significant prevalence of avoidable blindness should be encouraged to increase the content of ophthalmology in the undergraduate medical curriculum, with emphasis on community ophthalmology. It is further recommended that courses should also be provided for the reorientation of physicians and ophthalmologists to the community aspects of ophthalmology.

5. The IAPB should collect and distribute information on personnel needed and available for blindness prevention programmes, and techniques needed and available for use in these programmes. Among the technical problems requiring special attention are means of producing drugs and spectacles using locally available manpower and materials, adaptation of ophthalmic equipment for use in the field, and simplification of surgical methods.

6

Resource mobilization

Without resources of finance, personnel, and goodwill, no prevention of blindness programme can proceed. The following papers suggest how to mobilize those resources and how to seek assistance from local communities, non-governmental organizations, charitable foundations, and governmental agencies. The papers are followed by relevant recommendations made during the course of the assembly.

ECONOMIC JUSTIFICATION AND IMPLICATIONS FOR THE PREVENTION OF BLINDNESS
J. H. Costello

All of us know that programmes and strategies for the prevention of blindness have an economic cost and implication, and that those of us involved as planners, implementors, and humanitarians must convince donors—be they individuals, institutions, corporations, or governments—that their investment, whether $2 or $2 million, is justifiable.

Without a doubt, we are expert in pleading the case for blindness prevention on humanitarian grounds. For the past 70 years this has been, and continues to be, the central theme for the generation of resources for almost every operational institution represented within IAPB—whether indigenous, national, or international. It would never be appropriate to drop the human concern from our consciousness or our message. It is far too important, and is at the core of each organization's identity and purpose. However, while continuing to make the case for blindness prevention on humanitarian grounds, we must—if we are to achieve significant strides in blindness prevention on a broad scale—make the economic case as well.

In an era of shrinking resources amid vastly increasing health and development demands, we cannot reasonably expect continued, or much less expanded, investment on a substantial scale unless we can present policy and decision makers with hard data which pinpoint interventions that are justifiable, at least in terms of cost effectivness and, if possible, in terms of cost benefit. We must initiate the types of operational research—using research in its very broadest definition —which will result, not only in designing the methodologies and strategies for reaching large populations at risk with measurable impact, but which will produce reasonable economic indicators as well. We must, for example, be able to establish current costs for the delivery of services and project the recurring costs that are required over a reasonable period of time for the achievement of a targeted reduction of avoidable blindness in a given population. To the degree possible, these data should be linked to the cost to an individual, to a community, or to a nation of not investing in intervention strategies. All this is a formidable task for which little exists in the way of systematic data gathering and analyses. But the challenge must be met; the objectives have been set; and Helen Keller International (HKI) is taking the first steps.

I would like to take a moment briefly to review one or two important recommendations which were set forth by two important WHO task force meetings—the Planning Group on Research Priorities, which met at the Pan American Health Organisation (PAHO) in September 1979, and the Task Force Meeting on Economic Implications of Blindness Prevention, again held at PAHO in July 1980. The recommendations of these two groups are related because the methods suggested for reaching the largest number of people at the lowest possible per capita cost also provide keys to the development of replicable strategies for determining cost effectiveness.

Basically, it was recommended that various eye health care strategies be built into a selected number of primary health care system in different countries. In each, it would be important to mount studies to determine the degree of co-ordination required from the secondary and tertiary levels to maintain a continued, effective system of eye health care and prevention at the primary level. The measurement and analysis of the added costs at each level, it was suggested, should be built into the delivery systems, and the programme impact examined. Because of regional variations—notably the prevalence of disease, the state of the health infrastructure, population size and density, literacy rates—it appeared that detailed studies in about four different countries would be needed.

As a result of this thinking, HKI initiated, in 1981, the most ambitious and significant programme in its 67-year history. This involved the development and implementation of a carefully targeted programme aimed at integrating basic preventive eye care services, or primary eye care, into the delivery of primary health care in four developing countries. While the major aim is to develop reasonable strategies which will reach people at risk, and which can be readily replicated elsewhere, the programme has an economic objective as well. To the degree that it proves possible, we intend to measure at the very least, cost effectiveness, and, where and when possible, cost benefit too.

We envisage a long-term commitment in each country with programme operations being phased in over a 3-year period in Peru, Sri Lanka, Tanzania and, possibly, the Philippines with an initial 3-year budget of $3 million, jointly financed by USAID and HKI. The selection of these four countries is important because of the variables that will enable us to develop models relating to a wide range of disparate factors. To guide the planning and implementation process, HKI has established a task force which includes, in addition to ophthalmologists, public health specialists, and epidemiologists, a team of economists from Cornell University with solid experience in 'Third World' development.

The Peru programme after more than 2 years of planning began in December 1982, and programmes in Sri Lanka and Tanzania are scheduled to start in mid-1983. It will be apparent from the start that the emphasis is on cost effectiveness in that we will concentrate, at least initially, on the most readily avoidable causes of blindness—xerophthalmia and infectious eye diseases—where we can be seen to achieve the greatest impact in the shortest time.

There are still many issues that must be confronted before it can be demonstrated just how cost effective such programmes can be. For example, what direct and indirect costs should be entered into our equations? How can we be certain that the data provided are accurate? Should transfer payments and related start-up costs be amortized over a long period or be entirely separate from annual recurring costs? And, of course, valid baseline data must be collected before programme impact can be evaluated at determined intervals.

Perhaps the most difficult challenge will be to develop ways to measure cost benefit, because arbitrary values must be assigned to various outcomes for various persons at different life stages. The method we have proposed, for the moment, is based on valuing the income stream, the cost of hiring a service to be performed or the cost of a person's not being able to participate in an income-producing activity.

Many hurdles face us, and the task of gathering data covering a multiple of variables seems at times almost too complicated to achieve. But at HKI we have set in motion the wheels that will speed us to the goal of development of effective and useful methodologies for proving that the amount of blindness in a given country can be drastically reduced at reasonable cost—that our programmes can, in fact, be cost effective. It is no longer enough to say that blindness prevention is humane and that it is inexpensive, therefore funds should be committed. We are setting out to prove that no nation can afford not to take part.

AVAILABILITY OF AND NEED FOR DEVELOPMENT OF MULTINATIONAL RESOURCES WITHIN A REGION *R. Pararajasegaram*

Programmes for eye care delivery should ideally be based on national resources and self-reliance. However, this ideal is not, for the foreseeable future, within the reach of most countries in the Southern

Asia region because of the low priority generally given to health programmes in overall development plans. In addition, relatively insignificant support has been given, at least in the past, to the eye care component in health delivery.

The reasons for this state of affairs are not far to seek. Four of the countries included in the region fall into the category of what has been described by the United Nations as Least Developed Countries (LDCs). The countries are Bangladesh, Bhutan, the Maldives, and Nepal. The main criteria used by the United Nations to define an LDC are a very low income per person, low levels of adult literacy, and low output of manufactured goods. These four countries are also either land-locked, mountainous, prone to droughts or floods or have difficulties in communication. To quantify some of these criteria: per capita income is under $100 per annum, illiteracy is over 75 per cent, only half of all children even begin school, and only 16 per cent of the people's caloric requirements are met. About a third of their total population including two out of three children are undernourished.

The remaining countries in the region which include Burma, India, and Sri Lanka are 'Third World' countries, only a little better off than the LDCs. The need for resource mobilization is therefore obvious.

Resources

Trained personnel

National resources include ophthalmic personnel comprising opthalmologists, ophthalmic-trained medical officers, ophthalmic assistants, and other categories of health personnel trained to various levels of competence in the delivery of eye care. Though prevention of blindness programmes are a multisectoral and multidisciplinary effort and cannot be equated merely with the availability of ophthalmologists, nevertheless trained ophthalmologists are needed not only to work within their immediate discipline but also to provide wide ranging back-up services. They are required to provide secondary and tertiary level care as support for referral services with suitable training in management methodology, epidemiology, biostatistics, etc. They may be needed to serve as managers, survey directors, etc., in the implementation of the programmes.

All the countries in the region have a dearth of ophthalmologists. India, which is considered to be the best placed with about 5000 ophthalmologists, nevertheless shows a marked disparity of numbers between rural and urban areas. The remaining countries of the region, with a population of approximately 170 million, have between them about 150 ophthalmologists, and this again does not reflect the relative paucity in the rural areas. For instance, in Nepal, a population of 6 million in the western and far western region had no ophthalmologist till last year.

Ophthalmic assistants and technicians are a new concept in most countries of the region except Bangladesh, Burma, and India. Burma utilized ophthalmic assistants in their Trachoma Control Programme as far back as 1964. They were trained to perform lid surgery for entropion. The numbers of this grade of personnel now available in these three countries amount to approximately 150, 550, and 2000, respectively. Nepal has launched a training programme both locally in Nepal and also in institutions in India. Sri Lanka is launching an ophthalmic assistants' training programme in 1983. The Nepal programme has built into it the capacity to train 94 ophthalmic assistants.

With regard to other health care personnel, it is difficult to quantify the number of the medical and paramedical people already trained or to be trained in eye care. Such plans for appropriate personnel development are important components of the national programmes and are receiving top priority.

Ophthalmic beds

The availability of ophthalmic beds in a country determines to a large extent the turnover of surgical cases, especially cataract. In India, the number of eye beds is approximately 22 000. In the other countries put together, the total amounts to 3000. The shortfall in bed strength is partly met by the outreach programmes which include the use of mobile units, eye camps, base hospitals, etc.

Mobile units

Though mobile units have been in vogue in the Indian subcontinent for several decades, it is a relatively new modality of eye care delivery, particularly in sight restorative surgery, in Nepal, Burma, Sri Lanka, and the Maldives.

Community participation

The community and its active participation in the planning and implementation of programmes for eye care is an invaluable resource particularly at primary care levels. Comprehensive eye care with community involvement provides an infrastructure at grass roots level to tackle the many environmental, nutritional, and personal hygiene problems that underlie many of the causes of avoidable blindness. Eye health promotion through health education is a community activity of prime importance. Community participation is a vital component of outreach programmes such as mobile units and eye camps for treatment of the curably blind.

Non-governmental organizations

Several charitable organizations and trusts, including religious bodies, have been set up in countries of the region to support eye care activities.

These include hospital out-patient clinics, mobile units, school screening programmes, etc. There is a need for co-ordination of these efforts to ensure non-duplication and quality of service.

The national chapters of international organizations such as Rotary, Lions, Red Cross, and Jaycees, to name a few, have for several decades been active in sight preservation and restoration of vision programmes. Their support is an invaluable national and regional resource. Contributions by national governments, charitable and service organizations, and the community often provide the seed money for initiating programmes. These, in turn, attract funds from regional, bilateral, multilateral, and international sources once the feasibility and credibility of the project is established.

Technical co-operation among developing countries

At a regional level, an increasingly important resource is Technical Co-operation among Developing Countries (TCDC). This concept has found wide application in the field of blindness prevention in the Southern Asia region. India, with its highly trained manpower in institutions such as the Rajendra Prasad Centre for Ophthalmic Sciences, a WHO Collaborating Centre, the Sarojini Devi Eye Hospital, the Aravind Eye Hospital, and the Sitapur Hospital, to name a few, provide such technical co-operation. Besides undertaking the training of ophthalmologists and paramedical personnel from member countries of the region, specialists at these and other institutions have served as consultants in neighbouring countries both in assisting nationals in formulating plans of action and in evaluation of programmes. A recent development is the harnessing of such expertise in organizing sight restoration camps in countries like Sri Lanka, the Republic of Maldives, and possibly in Nepal to help clear the large backlog of avoidable blindness from cataract in these countries.

Budgeting

Budgeting should be a fundamental part of planning. This is based on the activities that are to be undertaken and the costing of those activities. The World Health Organization budgets on a biennial basis and budgeting takes place 2 years ahead.

Funding

The WHO affords technical co-operation to member states in each programme area. The financial implications of this may be met through:

(a) the regular country budget;
(b) the regular inter-country budget; and
(c) extra budgetary resources.

The amount of the regular country budget assigned to the prevention of blindness activities in each country depends on the political will generated and the commitment of the health planners. The ophthalmic lobby can influence this. For instance, the regular country budget for prevention of blindness activities in India has multiplied twenty-fold between 1982-3 and 1984-5 since prevention of blindness became a part of the government 20-point programme. The regular budget merely provides 'seed money' in most instances.

The regular inter-country budget provides funds that are used to finance programmes of a regional nature and the Regional office has some control over the apportioning of this in respect of the member states. It is utilized for the recruitment of consultants, for general educational activities, fellowships, and supplies of equipment.

Extra budgetary funds provide the bulk of the resources for the operation of the prevention of blindness programmes. These funds may be provided as finance or as supplies, etc., by other United Nations agencies such as the United Nations Development Programme (UNDP) and United Nations Children's Fund (UNICEF). On the other hand, private non-governmental foundations, trusts, etc., may contribute to the World Health Organization's voluntary fund for health promotion. This fund, set up in Geneva, channels contributions received to various programmes, through the regional offices which, in turn, allot these to different member states.

These contributions may be designated for prevention of blindness programmes in general or may be intended for a specific country. Examples of donors providing this type of support include the Japanese Shipbuilding Industry Foundation (JSIF), the Royal Commonwealth Society for the Blind, the Asian Foundation for the Prevention of Blindness, and for specific country funding the Norwegian and Dutch governments' development programmes.

Member states of WHO requiring funds are urged to prepare feasibile and credible projects relevant to the needs of their countries, not only in service delivery but also with regard to research. These project proposals, which should include detailed budgetary requirements, are then received by the respective regional office and submitted to the prevention of blindness programme in Geneva where they are catalogued and submitted to the meeting of donor agencies. Projects are likely to attract the attention of donors if they appear realistic and are in tune with present thinking and concepts of primary health care, community-oriented eye health care, and outreach eye health modes of delivery. Apart from the relevance of the proposals to local needs and conformity to the local socio-economic conditions, donor agencies also look at their cost effectiveness. Programmes that offer the greatest good, to the largest number, in perhaps, the shortest possible time, at the lowest cost, naturally are likely to be considered the most attractive.

In conclusion; the increased national awareness and the expressed political will and commitment to the cause of prevention and control of blindness and blinding diseases augurs well for the future of these programmes. With the funds that are likely to become increasingly available to the region from foundations and agencies who have already proved their concern, a decisive impact in breaking the link between blindness and population growth can be expected in the foreseeable future with an overall elimination of preventable and curable blindness. Such a policy has been described by the Director General of the World Health Organization as 'one of the most cost effective options in the whole contemporary range of world health policy'.

MOBILIZATION OF BILATERAL RESOURCES
A. T. Jenkyns

Many countries are already involved to a greater or lesser extent with the mobilization of bilateral resources. This type of assistance can be very large and very effective. It has many aspects including:

(a) financial—this is the prime component and is usually big and provides capital for buildings, equipment, and programmes;
(b) personnel—help with funding teams, etc.; and
(c) training at all levels.

In some western countries, international and national non-governmental organizations (NGOs) assist in the management of bilateral programmes on behalf of their governments. In other countries, government monies are channelled through national and international NGOs who have the ability to reach grass roots programmes, while governments sometimes cannot do this. In addition, of course, NGOs can attract funds from the citizens of their country and create a broader awareness of the needs of people in developing countries.

Because ophthalmic health care in any country, especially smaller ones, must be integrated ultimately into the country's overall health care programme, it is essential that the government of the country becomes involved in programmes through its Ministry of Health. Thus one side of the bilateral coin is already developed in many countries. The other side, linking up with the government of another country, may still have to be undertaken.

Sources of support

When an NGO such as Operation Eyesight Universal (OEU) is seeking sight restoration and blindness prevention programmes it is looking for an indigenous partner: a legal charitable entity that is undertaking or wants to undertake eye work—primarily for the poor. OEU welcomes proposals, for it never imposes a programme on an indigenous group; rather, it sets out to support a programme which has been presented by a local group and which will be administered by local people.

NGOs have especially useful roles to fulfil in providing support which may be overlooked by governments. They have an ability to focus on sectors, communities or programmes which may otherwise remain neglected.

Finally, Canadian Government assistance is moving toward a total aid programme by core countries and regions. This effort will incorporate bilateral, multilateral, and special programmes, commercial assistance, and will involve NGOs and other agencies.

THE ROLE OF PHILANTHROPY IN RESOURCE MOBILIZATION K. L. Stumpf

Philanthropy, like investment in securities, was once thought of as the peculiar domain of the very wealthy. The average citizen, dropping his coins in the plate at Sunday church, or paying his dues to the local parent-teacher association, or making his modest contribution to the Red Cross, has never thought of himself as a philanthropist. Yet, statistics show that the individual giver provides two-thirds or more of the total charitable funds raised in western countries, with the bulk of the funds coming from the lower-middle and middle economic groups.

Philanthropy in the developed countries, especially in the USA, is big business. Billions of dollars are contributed annually to charitable causes. Obviously, then, philanthropy is not an esoteric matter; it is of vital concern to all, whose work is to devise strategies which, so we hope, will enable the International Agency for the Prevention of Blindness to be more effective in achieving its objectives. We are, therefore, involved in a marketing process whether or not we are conscious of it. The issue is not whether or not we, as a non-profit-making organization, should get involved in marketing our cause, but rather how thoughtful we should be at it. Resources must be attracted, governments and people must be stimulated, patients and doctors must be motivated in the use and development of services. The designing of proper incentives is a key step in overcoming apathy or indifference and in promoting adequate financial support.

The concept of philanthropy is in the finest traditions of a democratic society. It is self-help voluntarily undertaken and given by private citizens, designed to complement, and in some instances, to outdo the role of government in the areas of health, welfare, education, and other fields of social service. By their very nature, philanthropic funds can be used to break new ground and to broaden horizons— goals frequently barred to government agencies. Under totalitarian forms of government, private philanthropy is non-existent. The state is considered to minister to all needs and so exacts maximum tribute from the citizens both financially and ideologically. There is no room under a dictatorship for new ideas other than those which are handed down by the ruling hierarchy.

But the very fact that a democratic society provides a hot-house atmosphere for private philanthropic effort to flourish, may itself sometimes create problems through sheer magnitude. Such difficulties are likely to be resolved through a combination of moderate and constructive government regulations, and a substantial amount of self-discipline and self-regulation by the giving public and the receiving agencies.

The role and function of philanthropy has undergone considerable changes in the past few decades. The support of those who cannot provide their own basic needs is now accepted as a government responsibility. No welfare department of any country or city is thought of or described as a philanthropic or charitable agency. It is rather an integral part of a network of protective services provided by law which includes social insurance, free hospital treatment, community health services, and so on. The community's taxing power is and should be the basic resources for meeting the fundamental needs of food, clothing, shelter, and personal care.

Modern philanthropy is, therefore, no longer primarily concerned or involved with 'support to the needy'. Modern philanthropy has instead a wider and equally important function to perform, and that is the provision of services and the support of research. Both of these objectives are fruitful in raising the level of human health and happiness. They may also relieve the community's financial burden. The philanthropic dollar, wisely spent, multiplies itself a thousand times in ultimate financial savings to the community as a whole. A modest grant of $25 000, made to a team of researchers in the area of blindness prevention, may save hundreds of thousands of dollars of the taxpayers' money. Therefore, the watchword of modern philanthropy is 'you have to spend money to save money'.

Charitable, non-profit-making organizations depend very much on the services and contributions of individual volunteers, donors, and philanthropic organizations. Volunteers include a variety of persons who feel a social responsibility to lend their time to agencies to help them carry on their work. Volunteers do not expect any payment other than appreciation. Many agencies have instituted special programmes to honour their volunteers and to give them a feeling of pride in their work.

Individual donors include wealthy people who may give substantial support to an agency and many other people who make small but thoughtful donations. The agency's director has the task of attracting and maintaining generous and loyal donors. To be effective, the director has to have a good understanding of the motivations of people for supporting his agency. Contributors include people who want to feel pride in their local community. The director, in addition to needing empathy with various groups of donors, must exhibit other skills. He must have a well organized approach to fund raising. He must be able to develop effective communication appeals that inspire people to contribute. He must follow up their contributions with acknowledgements and proposals for further involvement. His general aim is to create feelings in donors that they are worthwile supporters of a worthwhile cause.

The upkeep and development of philanthropic giving is essential because the welfare industry is a money-poor industry. Welfare is not produced and sold to consumers at a price covering its costs. Money is raised through public funds and private gifts to supplement the inadequate user charges.

Traditionally, non-profit organizations have not paid the kind of attention to the development and management of their financial resources that is found in most business establishments. This relative lack of concern goes unpenalized as long as their services are in high demand and funds are relatively easy to obtain. Today, the situation is different. Major sources of financial support are moderating their generosity at a time when the cost of living is rapidly increasing at all levels.

Therefore, an agency has to make sure that no potential source of funds is overlooked and that all contributing sources are producing at their maximum. Fund raising, therefore, must be viewed as a separate art, or in wider terms, as a marketing problem. Viewed as a marketing problem, the task is to analyse the level of current money flow from various sources and to consider ways to increase this flow. Ultimately, social service agencies must analyse their markets for funds as carefully as soap and car manufacturers analyse their markets for detergents and automobiles. This means developing models of fund-giving behaviour and determining the best way to increase the perceived benefits to the fund suppliers in return for their support.

If we are to advance beyond these general formulations, we must recognize that although the fund-raising problem is faced by all types of non-profit organizations, the structure of this problem varies greatly from one type to another.

It is indeed a creative challenge to select concepts and tools that are particularly appropriate for the marketing of a cause which protects and furthers the well-being of our fellow men and women. But there are hundreds of non-governmental and non-profit organizations striving to motivate the public to adopt a new cause, to alter beliefs, attitudes, values or the behaviour of targeted groups of the public. The National

Safety Council wants people to wear seat belts when driving. The American Anti-Cancer Society wants people to stop smoking. The National Organization of Women wants men to view women as their equals. And a fund-raising concept which works for churches may not be useful for hospitals.

The International Agency for the Prevention of Blindness promotes the setting up of blindness prevention programmes on a global scale. The agency provides a rich conceptual system for thinking through the problems of bringing about changes in the world's major blindness conditions and to transform world interest into world action. If, with the help of philanthropic giving, additional resources are to be mobilized, we need new innovative designs, methods of effective implementation and the control of programmes which aim to increase the acceptability of our objectives: to prevent people losing their sight because of poverty, ignorance, malnutrition, and lack of medical care and facilities.

In conclusion: a simple study of the world situation will bring to light a shocking variety of unmet human needs and suffering, among them needless, preventable blindness. These needs and problems exist in spite of the provisions made by the welfare state, the United Nations agencies and non-profit organizations. Many of these needs could be met by a revival of genuine philanthropy. The projects undertaken by the IAPB clearly show how many opportunities still exist for the philanthropist for helping people in distress. The true philanthropist is not satisfied with good intentions and warm regards but wants to respond to a need by action.

Responding and caring to a human need requires knowledge which we must provide. The person who cares wants to know for whom he cares, what the needs are, and what is conducive in bringing about the change in the lives of people who are ill, undernourished, poor, and homeless. The growing awareness on the part of philanthropy of the value of supplementary help will then be matched by a reawakening of social conscience in other sections of our world's communities which finds expression in a desire to give time, talents, and service in areas of human needs.

The philanthropist, who may also be called 'the good neighbour', was a very important person in Old Testament days. He was a very important person in the days of Christ, and he is still a very important person today. In fact, we see now more clearly than we did a few years ago that the philanthropist has a central, rather than a marginal role to play in helping to tackle the many human needs and problems of our time.

FUND RAISING W. Stein

It has been claimed that the existence and effectiveness of the International Agency for the Prevention of Blindness rests on three columns: personnel, finance, and commitment. In acknowledging and commending that statement I would like to add the following: while we are all convinced that 'personnel' and 'commitment' are interrelated, we rarely see the unity of 'finance' and 'commitment', particularly if we think in terms of raising the funds necessary for our activities.

I believe that fund raising cannot be guided simply by special techniques and commercial strategies. Fund raising, that is soliciting money from our fellow citizens, in fact has a great deal to do with commitment and ultimately rests on the principles of morals and ethics. We would all be very happy if und raising campaigns were unnecessary, if there was enough money available to finance our programmes to prevent blindness and other handicaps, to heal the sick, and to bring relief to the suffering. Unfortunately, this is not the case. Because of an invisible boundary around the globe, separating the rich from the poor, we will have to make continued efforts to bridge the gap between those two worlds for many years to come. Our activities are focused on countries which rank among the poorest in today's world, and in spite of all goodwill on the part of their governments, they will not be able to solve their problems without assistance from outside.

In past years governments in industrialized countries have made substantial funds available to the developing part of the world, but their contributions have only met a fraction of the actual needs. Economic recession and declining tax income will result in further reduction of their assistance. Consequently, funds have to be found from other sources, and this is the task of non-governmental agencies. As a representative of such an organization I am glad to testify to the fact that there is a vast reservoir of goodwill and readiness in our countries to help the 'distant neighbour'. It is the millions of pensioners, widows, college students, housewives, and ordinary people in the street, who care for others, and who are quite willing to share whatever they have with their needy fellow human beings throughout the world. They have responded—and I am sure they will continue to do so in the future—to our plea to share rather than to 'give' or to 'donate'. We must abolish the terms of 'giving' and 'receiving' and encourage the belief and principle of 'sharing'. It is not welfare that our world needs, but the solidarity of mankind!

But we must remember, these good people make sacrifices not in order to make our organizations grow: they want to see speedy results achieved by means of their contributions, they want to see action! A women who contributed $20 has a right to know that with her money, eyesight has been restored to another woman in a faraway corner of the world—she is unlikely to be interested in our world-wide strategies and 'global programmes'. To motivate her and other good-hearted people, we must observe certain fundamental rules, of which I outline just a few.

1. Slogans, such as 'Help the Blind' or 'Give to the Poor', cannot motivate a donor. An honest and plain presentation of the nature and extent of the problem, its causes, and consequences, is more likely to attract the attention of a donor than vague and ambiguous 'appeals for help'.
2. Presentations should refrain from employing techniques which could sarcastically be described as the 'pornography of suffering'. The illustration of human misery by horror pictures and exaggerated reports very often has adverse effects, because instead of encouraging potential donors it repels them. In spite of our knowledge of colossal poverty, need, and suffering, we must, in all our actions, observe human dignity and self-respect. All our endeavours must be guided (and this philosophy should be shared with the donor) by the conviction that we are helping a fellow human being.
3. We should give the donor the feeling that his contribution makes him a participant in our programme. He has a right to be informed of our plan of action, so that he can identify himself with our strategy and with the aims and objectives of our programmes.
4. It follows that the donor has a right to be informed about the progress of our activities at regular intervals, as he wants to know how his donation has been utilized. Experience has shown that regular reporting encourages donors to accept new commitments.

Fund raising is not a mere technical undertaking, but an action of solidarity, guided by a spirit of goodwill, understanding, and hope for mankind. In order to express and to exercise this conviction, we should mobilize all resources available, while at the same time being good stewards of the funds entrusted to us. We must use them wisely and economically, so that we are recognized as trustworthy partners by the people who so generously support us.

THE DEVELOPMENT OF GOVERNMENTAL AND INTER-GOVERNMENTAL RESOURCES
Dorina de Gouvêa Nowill

The importance of directly involving communities in programmes concerned with assisting people who are physically or sensorially handicapped is increasingly being recognized by government authorities and health programme organizers. Indeed, such programmes will only flourish as a result of community interest and participation, preceded by an awakening consciousness of their relevance.

In a number of developing countries, existing governmental campaigns for the prevention of blindness have been created as a direct consequence of community participation, and today they are part of regularly planned official activities.

The importance of setting up prevention of blindness programmes has been recognized in many countries of the world. Such programmes exist at federal, state, and local levels. Because of the complexity surrounding the whole subject it is essential that formal responsibility for the establishment and maintenance of prevention of blindness programmes should rest with government agencies. Without this official support very little will be done, and almost nothing of a concrete and lasting nature will be accomplished. Government support is necessary to ensure that programmes of this sort, especially in poorer and less developed countries, are incorporated into primary health care programmes. Prevention of blindness activities need to be included as a part of measures concerned with basic sanitation, an adequate supply of safe water, immunization against major infectious diseases, nutritional programmes, and educational measures concerned with prevention and control of disease.

Unfortunately, notwithstanding the undeniable need for governments to be involved in blindness prevention activities within their own countries, official priorities are often geared towards other objectives. In these circumstances, financial support, basic resources, and necessary personnel are difficult to obtain.

Where a government requests technical assistance in setting up a prevention of blindness programme, intergovernmental agencies of a regional or an international character can play an important role in assisting that country in its efforts. Such agencies are able to provide the required technology and can help governments in establishing the necessary strategies.

Basic proposals

Every developing country, whatever the level of development, should channel some resources to undertake at least basic activities for blindness prevention including annual treatment of eye diseases in individual patients. Since there is usually a shortage of funds for specific separate health campaigns, primary eye care should be inserted in basic education, basic health care, nutritional, and basic sanitation programmes.

Measures specifically oriented towards the integration of prevention of blindness in such programmes depend very much on information being available regarding the extent of the problems and the existence of a means for inexpensive and integrated action. In the early phase of a programme, when such matters are being considered, the co-operation of non-governmental organizations (NGOs) such as the International Agency for the Prevention of Blindness (IAPB) and the

World Council for the Welfare of the Blind (WCWB), as well as organizations of blind persons such as the International Federation of the Blind can be instrumental in ensuring the programme starts from a firm base. These organizations often have national or regional representatives who are well placed to liaise with both local private agencies and those at government level. It is essential that such representatives should be kept fully informed of policies and strategies at all time. Firm and decisive interest shown by international agencies will also guarantee the closest co-operation of private organizations which have already been involved with prevention of blindness activities for many years.

When considering the broader implications of prevention of blindness campaigns it is important to recognize the crucial role played by the WHO through its Programme Advisory Group on the Prevention of Blindness. Furthermore, the effectiveness of its work is enhanced through close liaison with governmental and non-governmental organizations.

Co-ordination of all the interested agencies is vital. It is possible that this could be achieved by creating an international agency co-ordination body which would be responsible for planning and implementation of programmes, as well as training of personnel in basic eye care procedures. It would work through the recommendations made by the WHO Programme Advisory Group. Through this co-ordinating body, activities would be better controlled, and useful initiatives undertaken. For example, UNESCO, with close co-operation from the WHO and UNICEF should encourage governments to ensure that school teachers at preschool and elementary grade levels should have, within their training curriculum, an element concerned with basic eye care procedures. Similar approaches could be made to other agencies who have a potential role to play in combating preventable or remediable blindness including the International Labour Organization, the Organization of American States, and the regional offices of international organizations.

Only well co-ordinated action will provide the necessary means for effective programmes of blindness prevention. It is the only route to reach the WHO goal of 'Health for All by the Year 2000'.

COMMUNICATIONS, PUBLICITY, AND PUBLIC RELATIONS *Jean Wilson*

In the four years since the last Assembly 1978, there has been a considerable flow of publications, most of them resulting from the WHO Programme Advisory Group on the Prevention of Blindness. These are now being augmented by publications from the collaborating centres and research organizations. The IAPB has participated in many of these publications, and itself has developed three levels of communication.

At the first level we have the book *World blindness and its prevention* which incorporated material presented at the First General Assembly in 1978. It was the first in a series of books planned to follow the IAPB's four-yearly assemblies. These books, of which this is the second, aim to be authoritative reviews on policies and strategies and are directed to planners, legislators, development economists, prevention of blindness practitioners, and medical students.

At the second level, we have the journal *Vision*, imaginatively conceived and developed by Dr Arthur Lim and his editorial board, and impressively published in Singapore. This journal is directed primarily to ophthalmic surgeons, but I know that Dr Lim's intention is that its content in future should be broadened to attract a multidisciplinary readership.

At the third level, and designed especially for our own readership, are the newsletters, of which the most comprehensive was published as background to this Assembly.

This is, I think, the right framework and, so far, the Agency has succeeded, at surprisingly modest cost, in maintaining these publications. For the present, they are mainly the work of headquarters and the South-East Asia Regional Committee, but it would surely be desirable to aim for a much broader participation and coverage, perhaps with a newsletter in each region and bulletins on specific disease categories modelled on the excellent xerophthalmia bulletin to which Dr Pirie gives such devoted service. Funds are limited, but we have found that publications of the quality I have described can often be promoted at little cost to central funds. The question should be examined of financial sponsorship by companies which have a legitimate interest in the prevention of blindness. For example, by insurance companies and the manufacturers of drugs and equipment, though of course, such sponsorships should not be accepted if it implies any limitation on editorial policy.

Publicity and public relations are essential to the whole work of the Agency. In the broadest sense it is necessary for what we used to call its climate-changing role and, more specifically, for publicizing the achievements of model projects, the state of the art and, the always essential, fund raising.

The aim of an IAPB public relations programme is to achieve national and international awareness of the problem of avoidable blindness, and of the comparatively simple measures by which it can be tackled. At the international level this should be the constant task of the Agency's headquarters, working in co-operation with the WHO, UNICEF, and the international members. Regionally, it should be a function of the regional committee collaborating with the public information officers of regional United Nations organizations. Nationally, it should be a task for the national committees in liaison with national ministries and with the national representatives of United Nations organizations and professional bodies.

Should the Agency itself now work towards the establishment of a publicity bureau with one of its officers specifically assigned to this? Might there not be a publicity officer attached to each regional office and a public relations officer in each national committee? We achieved something very like this in the year when prevention of blindness was the theme of the World Health Day. I am sure we could again rely on the collaboration of the information departments of the UN agencies and of governments. Doctors look, with understandable misgiving, at publicity campaigns and fund raising, but the welfare organizations for the blind do not have that inhibition, and perhaps this is a direction in which an invaluable contribution to the Agency could be made by the blind welfare organizations which already have well-established publicity and public relations departments in North America, Europe, Hong Kong, Japan, and Australia. Publications must be readable and every communication must speak to its particular audience.

We hear so much about appropriate technology, but it will have little impact without appropriate communication. At one level, the prevention of blindness is a matter of precise, scientific communication, but at another, and probably more important level, it concerns public motivation.

The message of IAPB is basically simple: that most causes of avoidable blindness can be prevented by inexpensive action. We will have got that message across when people talk about it, not just in government offices, but in the market-place. Only the elite few can identify with abstract statistics about mankind—'that 100 000 blind people had sight-restoring operations in India last year'—we accept as good news, but we are not involved. 'When the bandages were removed from his eyes, young Krishna stretched out his fingers to grasp a handful of light.' Immediately, we are with that child, experiencing with him the wonder of seeing for the first time.

At the level of public motivation, the prevention of blindness needs to call on all the available resources of the media and to make effective use of audio-visual aids. Many hours of video tapes, and an impressive number of photographs and slides have been accumulated by members of the IAPB on prevention of blindness activities. These graphic pictures can be used to enlist public support. One good picture can save an hour of talk and can power a fund-raising project. It would be useful if each national delegation could regularly provide, both to the regional chairman and to headquarters, a few photographs of publishable quality.

As well as using the media, and visual aids, we may consider borrowing the techniques of the entertainment industry. An excellent example of this was recently instanced in the West Indies where, to promote a rubella immunization programme, a calypso was concocted. The first words go like this:

> Why all dis mystification
> Bout dis ding called immunization.
> It means— if you're going out with a fella
> Make sure you've had your rubella.

RECOMMENDATIONS

Participants at the Assembly of the IAPB agreed the following recommendations for the mobilization of resources.

1. Prevention of blindness programmes must be fully integrated into the primary health care system of each country, so that full use can be made of existing health care resources and activities. In this way, the expense of blindness prevention can be held to a minimum, and blindness prevention activities can be better justified to cost-conscious governments and other possible contributors of resources.
2. Information and, if possible, publications should be developed to document the cost-effectiveness of blindness prevention programmes. Such materials can be used to assure both official decision makers and private donors that contributions for the prevention of blindness will yield economic as well as humanitarian benefits.
3. The IAPB and its member organizations should improve their communications and publicity efforts. A book summarizing the presentations and deliberations of the Second General Assembly should be published;[1] the journal *Vision* should be continued with expanded readership; an IAPB newsletter should be published regularly. In addition, IAPB regional committees should be encouraged to retain their own public affairs officers and to publish regular newsletters.
4. The IAPB and its member organizations should extend their appeal for funds to corporations and individuals in all countries in order to increase the resources available for sight conservation and blindness prevention activities.
5. The IAPB should intensify its efforts to make ophthalmologists aware of the international effort to reduce the toll of avoidable blindness; IAPB should maintain a roster of ophthalmologists willing to work for a year or longer in developing countries, and should put these individuals in touch with countries or international organizations needing their services.

---

[1] This book, in fact, results from that recommendation.

Epilogue
Carl Kupfer

Dr Carl Kupfer, Director of the National Eye Institute, USA was elected as the second President of the International Agency for the Prevention of Blindness at the Second General Assembly of the Agency in October 1982. His acceptance speech provides the epilogue for this book.

As I look back on the Second General Assembly of the International Agency for the Prevention of Blindness, I find myself recalling a perception which Dr Robert Muller expressed in his keynote speech (see Chapter 1). He spoke about the fact that we all live on one planet: a living, concerned, and caring planet. I think the IAPB, and the participants in the Assembly reflected the sense of universal commitment that Dr Muller conveyed so well. There was an evident collegial spirit among the people from different countries and professions who have taken up the cause of preventing blindness.

More than anyone else, Sir John Wilson has been responsible for fostering that spirit. He has been the inspiration for the Agency, and we are indebted to him for guiding it into its current activist role. In his eight years as Agency president, he has alerted leaders of countries, officials of the World Health Organization, and decision-makers in the private and non-governmental sector to the vast needs and opportunities that exist in the field of blindness prevention. Also, he has focussed their attention on the need to make prevention of blindness programmes an integral part of all health care programmes.

In all the undertakings of the Agency, we must continue what Sir John has begun. We must considerably expand and strengthen the activities that link governments, international organizations, non-governmental organizations, and commited individuals in their efforts to prevent blindness. Attention must also be paid to cultivating grass roots support for the Agency, because a broad base of support is essential for any organization that hopes to flourish and grow.

In particular, we must intensify our efforts to mobilize resources for blindness prevention programmes. These resources are already in existence, but to secure them we must mount even more persuasive arguments than we have in the past. Our chances of doing this will be greatly increased if we can accomplish two outstanding tasks. One of these was identified by Dr Muller in his keynote address. It is to develop more precise data on the incidence, prevalence, causes, and costs of blindness so that we can better quantify the problems that we seek to solve. The second task is one that is always very difficult. That is to identify our priorities. We must define our priorities over both the short term and the long term, and we must express our goals in economic as well as humanitarian terms. Once we have done this, I believe that we will be in a position to make the most effective case possible on behalf of blindness prevention and to mobilize the resources that are required.

I expect that over the next few years there will be an acceleration in the rate of progress in blindness prevention programmes. We will make successes like those reported at the Assembly occur more rapidly, and I think the Agency will play a very important role as a stimulus for progress.

Ultimately, the challenge that we must strive to meet is the one expressed in the World Health Organization's slogan, 'Health for All by the Year 2000'. I am convinced that prevention of blindness programmes can meet that deadline if we maintain our determination and adopt effective medical and economic strategies. We can reduce avoidable blindness significantly, not just by the year 2000, but even before that. Large-scale victory will then be a reality in our battle against blindness.

Supplements

A. WHO COLLABORATING CENTRES FOR THE PREVENTION OF BLINDNESS

Eleven centres around the world are working in collaboration with the WHO and with each other in a concerted effort to prevent avoidable blindness. The provisional objectives already accepted by the centres which they will pursue to the best of their abilities, within the limits of their own programmes and budgetary constraints, include: active participation in development activities for the prevention of blindness; providing facilities for the training of personnel at different professional levels; conducting applied field research; fostering a multidisciplinary approach to the promotion of eye health and the delivery of eye care to all; collecting and distributing relevant information; providing on request the advisory services and expertise which might be required.

WHO Collaborating Centre	Director
AFRO	
Institut d'Ophtalmologie tropicale de l'Afrique, B.P. 248, Bamako, Mali.	Dr. P. Vingtain
AMRO	
International Center for Epidemiologic and Preventive Ophthalmology, The Wilmer Institute, 600 N. Wolfe Street, Baltimore, Maryland 21205, USA.	Dr A. Sommer
National Eye Institute, National Institutes of Health, Bethesda, Maryland 20014, USA.	Dr C. Kupfer
Eye & Ear Hospital Dr Rodolfo Robles V, National Committee for the Blind and Deaf, Guatemala City, Guatemala.	Dr L. Figueroa
Department of Ophthalmology, Santo Toribio de Mogrovejo Hospital, Ancash 1271, Lima, Peru.	Dr F. Contreras

WHO Collaborating Centre	Director
Francis I. Proctor Foundation for Research in Ophthalmology University of California, San Francisco, California 94143, USA.	Dr C. R. Dawson*
Serviço de Oftalmologia Sanitária, Secretaria de Estado da Saude, Av. Dr Enéas de Carvalho Aguiar No. 188, 8° Andar, Caixa Postal 8027, Sao Paulo, S.P. 05403, Brazil.	Dr O. Monteiro de Barros

EURO

Department of Preventive Ophthalmology, (International Centre for Eye Health), Institute of Ophthalmology, University of London, 27/29 Cayton Street, London, EC1V 2PD, UK.	Professor B. R. Jones*
Department of Viral and Allergic Eye Diseases, Helmholtz Research Institute of Ophthalmology, Sadovaja-Chernogriazslakaj 14/19, Moscow 103064, USSR.	Dr K. V. Trutneva†

SEARO

Dr Rajendra Prasad Centre for Ophthalmic Sciences, All-India Institute of Medical Sciences, Ansari Nagar, New Delhi 110016, India.	Professor M. Mohan

WPRO

Department of Ophthalmology, Juntendo University School of Medicine, 3-1-3 Hongo Bunkyo-ku, Tokyo, 113 Japan.	Professor A. Nakajima

*WHO Collaborating Centre for the Prevention of Blindness and Trachoma.
†WHO Collaborating Centre for the Prevention of Blindness Caused by Infectious Eye Diseases.

B. INTERNATIONAL NON-GOVERNMENTAL ORGANIZATIONS

The following NGOs make significant contributions to regional and national prevention of blindness programmes, and are affiliated to IAPB. They work closely with the WHO Programme Advisory Group on the Prevention of Blindness, government agencies, other voluntary organizations, and with each other.

The Asian Foundation for the Prevention of Blindness

The Foundation aims to participate in programmes throughout Asia, which break the link between blindness and population growth, in the hope that over the next decades preventable blindness in Asia will be reduced by half. Whilst the area of operation includes all countries in Asia, the governing body of the Foundation will base its decision as to which countries in Asia shall, from time to time, benefit through the Foundation's activities, upon the interest or preference of its main donors, inter-country relationships, and upon the assessment of priorities and opportunities. It will concentrate on those diseases which cause most of the blindness in Asia and for the control of which there exists an adequate technology which can be delivered at an acceptable level of cost effectiveness.

Hong Kong was chosen as the seat of the Foundation because of its strategic position as a crossroad of trade and culture, its extensive communications network, its scientific and economic resources as well as the managerial skill necessary to support a regional humanitarian foundation.

The Foundation sees its role in relation to regional and national programmes which are already in operation throughout Asia. However, because of the immense size of the problem, the Foundation is not in a position to tackle any major blindness prevention projects on its own and will, therefore, work in partnership with WHO, and well established national and/or international non-governmental agencies linked to the International Agency for the Prevention of Blindness, which have adequate manpower, research facilities, and field experience in the country where a project is to be undertaken. This, however, does not exclude the financing of smaller projects by the Foundation on its own initiative.

Since its inception in October 1981 the Foundation has been actively involved in blindness prevention programmes in Bangladesh, China, India, Indonesia, and Korea. The Foundation has, furthermore, supported and facilitated training programmes of ophthalmologists from Asia, and has enabled a number of ophthalmologists to participate at international conferences in the United States and Hong Kong.

Hong Kong and Singapore are not within the target areas of the Foundation. The prevalence of blindness in these two places is remarkably low and both areas have their own local or national bodies dealing with blindness and blindness prevention.

The Asian Foundation is aware that blindness prevention requires a multidisciplinary effort involving the ophthalmologist for treatment, the optometrist for the application of special aids, the health worker to assist the family, the patient to utilize community resources and cope with practical problems, the vocational rehabilitation counsellor to evaluate skills, to plan placement, self-employment or workshop programmes, and a corps of community volunteers to co-ordinate and stimulate project participation.

If the Asian Foundation is to mobilize additional resources for prevention of blindness projects, it is imperative that such programmes are effectively planned, implemented, and controlled. Responding and caring to a human need requires knowledge which must be provided. The donors who care want to know whom they care for, what the needs are, and what is conducive in bringing about the changes in the life of people whose blindness can be prevented or cured.

Further information from: Asian Foundation for the Prevention of Blindness, 33 Granville Road, Kowloon Road, Kowloon, Hong Kong.

The Christoffel-Blindenmission

Christoffel-Blindenmission—CBM as it is popularly known—is an inter-denominational Christian organization, committed to bringing hope to blind and otherwise handicapped people all over the world.

Named in honour of Pastor Ernst Christoffel, who worked among blind and handicapped people in the Middle East from 1908–55, CBM has grown rapidly in the past 25 years and is now reaching out to 90 countries in Asia, Africa, Latin America, and Oceania. CBM operates from Bensheim, West Germany, assisted by regional offices in Tiruchirapalli, India (for South-East Asia), Penang, Malaysia (for East Asia), Nairobi, Kenya (for Africa), Santa Cruz, Bolivia (for South America), and Port-au-Prince, Haiti (for Central America and the Caribbean).

These offices, in turn, have engaged the services of expert personnel in the fields of ophthalmology and optometry, education and rehabilitation, who guide, counsel, and advise in all decision-making processes. In contrast with other similar organizations, CBM has refrained from establishing and implementing its own programmes overseas. Instead, CBM supports national activities of churches, missions, and voluntary agencies in developing countries. The support is manifold: financial aid to cover operational expenses, provision of equipment, drugs, medicines, and instruments; but even more important, the secondment of expert personnel (at present 190 workers), who help to plan and carry out programmes for those who are sick and disabled.

The required funds for CBM's extensive services are raised entirely from hundreds of thousands of individual donors in Germany and some other European countries. In recent years, branch offices known as 'Christian Blind Mission International' were established in USA, Canada, and Australia, in order to motivate more donors in those parts of the world. Roughly 50 per cent of last year's annual income of US$25 million was sent for medical/ophthalmic programmes, whereas the other half was distributed among partners catering to the educational and rehabilitational needs of disabled people and, in particular, those who are blind.

While assisting partners in overseas at grass-roots level, CBM also contributes to international efforts in the battle against blindness. CBM has made contributions to research on onchocerciasis, xerophthalmia, and glaucoma. CBM has also helped to establish the International Agency for the Prevention of Blindness (in partnership with the Royal Commonwealth Society for the Blind), and co-operates with internationally recognized organizations such as Helen Keller International Inc. of USA, and Operation Eyesight Universal of Canada. For its manifold activities in this specific field, CBM is recognized as a non-governmental partner by WHO, UNICEF, UNHCR, and the World Council for the Welfare of the Blind.

Further information from: Christoffel-Blindenmission, Nibelungenstr. 124, D-6140 Bensheim 4, West Germany.

Foresight

The Overseas Aid Subcommittee of the Australian National Council of and for the Blind (ANCB), which was the vehicle for the channelling of funding for the Bangladesh project (see p. 45) has now been separately constituted into an independent organization called 'Foresight'—Australian Overseas Aid and Prevention of Blindness Organization. This non-governmental organization has tax-free privileges and has been recognized by the Australian Government.

Foresight has a number of projects, these are:

(a) training of doctors and paramedics to perform eye surgery in Bangladesh;
(b) building a new eye training complex in Bangladesh;
(c) supplying Port Moresby with equipment and library materials;
(d) starting eye departments in Port Moresby Hospital;
(e) assisting with the establishment of ophthalmology at Goroka, particularly with the fitting-out of the eye department;
(f) equipping and assisting in the establishment of eye departments in other centres in Papua New Guinea; and
(g) training of South Pacific field-workers in rehabilitation.

The aims of Foresight are to prevent and cure and, where this is not possible, to rehabilitate blind persons. The long-term aim is to improve ophthalmologic services to prevent blindness.

All these projects are supported by the government through the Australian Government Assistance Bureaux. Foresight raises portions of its funds through other aid organizations and members of ANCB, however, now Foresight benefits from the grant in tax deductibility it is planned to mount a separate fund-raising programme.

Further information from: Professor F. A. Billson, Department of

Clinical Ophthalmology, Sydney Eye Hospital, Sir John Young Crescent, Woolloomooloo, NSW 2011, Australia.

Helen Keller International

Helen Keller International (HKI) views world blindness as a public health problem. In order to make the greatest impact possible, we have given highest priority to the prevention of nutritional and infectious blindness, for it is in those areas that simple, inexpensive technology can be put to work. At the same time, by engaging in the rehabilitation and education work that prompted the founding of this agency 68 years ago, HKI continues its efforts to prepare people who are already blind for independent, productive lives.

Our attention is directed to the 'Third World', where conditions of impoverishment foster eye disease and where services are lacking or inadequate.

HKI's aim, in nations that invite our assistance, is provision of efficient, low-cost community-based care that can be sustained long after HKI consultants depart. A precondition of our intervention is the existence of at least a skeleton health care network that extends into the grass-roots level. We begin with small-scale geographically limited programmes in which methods for surveying disease prevalence, training personnel, delivering care, and evaluating effects can be tested quickly and replicated easily. Ideally, this effort will result in broad access to comprehensive eye-related care within the nation's primary health care system, with appropriate referrals made to secondary and tertiary medical centres.

Because countries vary in health care structures and rates of eye disease, HKI has no pat formula for its activities. Current work in ten nations shows a flexible approach determined by local conditions.

Bangladesh

Assistance to national nutritional blindness prevention programme reaching 60 per cent of the country's 20 million preschool-age children: vitamin-A-capsule distribution, programme assessment; nation-wide survey of nutritional blindness.

Fiji

Integrated education of blind students; community-based rehabilitation for blind adults; nation-wide survey of causes of blindness to assess eye care needs.

Haiti

Targeted distribution through 80 per cent of the nation's health establishments of vitamin-A-capsules to children at risk and lactating mothers; training health workers in eye care; nutrition education; surveillance of xerophthalmia cases.

India

Rehabilitation of the rural blind in Tiruchirapalli district in co-operation with Christoffel Blindenmission.

Indonesia

Vitamin A capsule distribution to 8.5 million children from April 1982 to March 1983; study of different capsule delivery systems in Aceh province; exploration of vitamin-A fortification of monosodium glutamate; extension of education of blind children to 200 villages; counselling parents of blind babies; nutrition education; non-formal education of the rural blind.

Malawi

Feasibility study of nutritional blindness prevention programme in the Lower Shire Valley, with the WHO and other blindness prevention agencies.

Peru

Introduction of primary eye care in three rural areas with a combined population of two million and in Lima shantytowns; disease prevalence surveys, training health providers, provision of instructional materials, and clinic equipment.

Philippines

Rehabilitation of the rural blind in seven of that nation's 13 regions.

Sri Lanka

Selection of demonstration sites for the introduction of primary eye care to the health care systems.

Tanzania

Feasibility study for primary eye care in the Dodoma regions, where an estimated 60 per cent of the population suffers from trachoma.

An additional aspect of HKI's work is building acceptance and support for blindness-related programmes. In our efforts to educate policymakers and the general public, we plan to augment humanitarian arguments with hard data that show the cost-effectivness and cost-benefits of our work.

A final note: it is self-evident that the battle against world blindness cannot be fought with traditional ophthalmology and rehabilitation alone. General development, particularly in agriculture and sanitation, is an essential weapon. To do our job, HKI not only joins forces with like-minded agencies, we seek alliances with organizations engaged in creating the climate in which our work will thrive.

Further information from: Helen Keller International, 15 West Sixteenth Street, New York 10011, USA.

International Eye Foundation

The humanitarian and development assistance programmes of the International Eye Foundation (IEF) are based on a philosophy dedicated to helping others to help themselves.

At the request of governments, the IEF provides technical assistance in determining the cause, extent, and resources available to treat blinding eye disease. With this information in hand, a practical, affordable national programme is developed with the government, stressing an integrated primary health care approach to provide curative and preventive eye-health-care delivery systems appropriate to the needs and resources of the country.

Drawing on the experience gained in over 20 years of helping others to help themselves, the IEF continued its progressive expansion of assistance activities during the past fiscal year, 1 July 1981 to 30 June 1982.

New dimensions were added in the efforts to relieve the suffering of the over 40 million blind people in the world and to reduce the dramatic increases in avoidable blindness. The IEF enlarged on its joint efforts with the World Health Organization and the governments of many countries. While continuing the highly successful programmes in specific countries, collaborative programmes were developed, joining neighbouring countries in shared programmes to combat blindness.

Full-time IEF staff, augmented by volunteer eye specialists, sponsored by the IEF and the Society of Eye Surgeons, continued long-term programmes in Honduras, Puerto Rico, St. Lucia, Kenya, Egypt, and Haiti. New programmes were begun in Guinea, Saudi Arabia, Malawi, Ecuador, and the Dominican Republic. Working in collaboration with the World Health Organization and other international agencies, assistance was given in the countries of Botswana, Malawi, Lesotho, Zimbabwe, Zambia, and Swaziland to evaluate the cause and extent of blinding eye disease. Country-specific programmes against blindness were developed, and a central training facility developed in Malawi to train health workers from these countries in the field of eye health care and blindness prevention.

Over 3600 auxiliary health workers, nurses, clinical officers, medical assistants, and their instructors were trained in the recognition, treatment or appropriate referral of patients suffering from eye disease. In order to help meet the demand for increased speciality eye services to prevent blindness and restore sight, 20 foreign physicians were given additional training in IEF-sponsored basic science and advanced speciality training courses. Thirty-four US eye specialists served abroad as short-term Visiting Professors and Surgeons, and nine served in full-time positions. Six certified ophthalmic technicians and nurses served in various developing countries. This impressive list of volunteers accounts for direct sight-saving and sight-restoring care for over 400 000 patients. Over 4000 major and minor surgical operations were performed by IEF staff during this period of time.

Foundations were laid for closer co-operation with other international organizations dedicated to blindness prevention and treatment in developing countries. By co-ordination of activities, our various complementary activities will be made far more effective and efficient.

Further information from: International Eye Foundation, 7801 Norfolk Avenue, Bethesda, Maryland 20814, USA.

International Glaucoma Association

The object of the International Glaucoma Association (IGA) is the preservation of sight by support for the improvement of resources for the early recognition, and for the highest standard of treatment of glaucoma.

Following the introduction in 1970 at the King's College Hospital Glaucoma Centre in London, of a computerized system of management designed to improve the care of glaucoma patients, it became clear that many patients had so little understanding of the disease that they were unable to co-operate in their treatment. Exploratory meetings between doctors and patients at the hospital revealed that many of the patients, who now number more than 1300, were very keen to meet eye specialists and fellow patients informally, so that problems could be more fully discussed. Many patients were also enthusiastic to improve the obviously limited resources available for investigation and treatment, and to encourage research into the many problems of glaucoma. During one of these meetings in 1974, and at the request of the patients themselves, the Glaucoma Association was formed, and a Council of officers appointed. The King's College Hospital Glaucoma Centre had already made contact with similar centres abroad, and indeed had patients in many other countries, and as glaucoma is a world-wide problem the name was changed to the International Glaucoma Association with the aim of co-operating with those in other countries who have the same objectives. Autonomous sections are being formed in India, South Australia, and Queensland, and are being considered in other countries. The IGA has developed its links widely by representative membership of the International Agency for the Prevention of Blindness, and affiliation with the International Glaucoma Congress of the American Society of Contemporary Ophthalmology.

The Association offers patients, doctors, opticians, optometrists, and all those interested in preventing blindness from glaucoma, a forum for the exchange of ideas as well as the opportunity to campaign actively for greater governmental recognition of the need for more resources to improve the detection of glaucoma and its treatment throughout the world. It must be emphasized that the disease responds much better to treatment if detected at an early stage.

The IGA holds an Annual General Meeting and discussion forums, and periodically organizes symposia. It also issues a newsletter and information booklets. There is a Scientific Section advising upon the medical problems of glaucoma, and in addition the Association helps to support clinical research projects.

By spreading information about glaucoma and by stimulating the greater provision of resources for early detection and careful management, the International Glaucoma Association aims to reduce as widely as possible, the needless misery caused by glaucoma blindness.

Further information from: International Glaucoma Association, Kings College Hospital, Denmark Hill, London SE5 9RS, England.

Operation Eyesight Universal

Founded in Calgary, Canada, in 1963 Operation Eyesight Universal (OEU) now reaches out helping hands to people in 16 of the world's developing nations. Just a handful of businessmen responded to a call to help one programme in 1963; today, thousands of people are involved in Canada and in three other continents. The organization, run by volunteers until 1977, is involved in programmes of sight restoration of the curably blind, and in projects of blindness prevention in some of the world's most economically depressed nations. In 1963 funds were provided to restore sight to 148 people. During 1981 OEU teams treated 673 741 people for a whole variety of eye problems, this was in addition to the figures quoted above. Mobile Eye Units are provided for a number of the projects and several ophthalmic hospitals have been built and/or expanded through OEU funds. Through the OEU Institute of Ophthalmology, part of the Kasturba Medical College at Manipal in the Indian State of Karnataka, ophthalmologists are being trained at postgraduate level. An ophthalmic paramedic training programme in Peru is also funded by OEU.

Operation Eyesight Universal also enjoys a very good relationship with the Government of Canada through the Canadian International Development Agency (CIDA), and several provincial governments. The Royal Commonwealth Society for the Blind has recognized OEU as a Commonwealth partner. It is also recognized by the Canadian Ophthalmological Society, the Canadian National Institute for the Blind and the Canadian Council of the Blind. OEU is also a member of the IAPB and an Associate Member of the World Council for the

Welfare of the Blind. OEU is a registered Canadian charitable corporation. During 1983 it will be funding 65 development projects.

Further information from: Operation Eyesight Universal, P.O. Box 123, Station 'M', Calgary, Alberta, Canada T2P 2H6.

The Royal Commonwealth Society for the Blind

The RCSB was founded in 1950 on the initiative of British and Commonwealth governments and with the active co-operation of national organizations for the blind, to prevent blindness and to provide education, rehabilitation, and employment for an estimated 15 million blind people in Commonwealth countries. In this the Society works with regional organizations, national governments, and with its national affiliated organizations in 28 Commonwealth countries.

Since 1970, medical teams sponsored by the Society have restored sight to more than a million blind people and treated over 10 million for various eye disorders that could have led to blindness.

Increasingly RCSB is providing essential medical supplies, sponsoring research, and training doctors and auxiliary workers. Nevertheless, amongst the Commonwealth's 15 million blind there are at least 6 million whose sight could be restored by inexpensive cataract surgery in eye camps.

The Society is now undertaking, in partnership with the Government of India, a major effort against blinding malnutrition—the world's largest destroyer of children's eyes. In India and Bangladesh each year some 65 000 babies needlessly go blind from this cause. Pilot projects and research in this field have shown that the sight of a child can be saved at minimal cost.

To provide education for as many as possible of the Commonwealth's 500 000 blind children, the Society helps to promote programmes of open education, as well as working with schools for the blind throughout Africa, Asia, and the Caribbean. The programme is also involved with training teachers and providing educational supplies. During the past 4 years RCSB has provided over 10 000 kits of essential braille equipment for the poorest children in the Commonwealth. Many talented scholars have also received higher education, in which some have already achieved outstanding academic success.

During recent years many blind adults have been the victims of economic depression. The Society aims to give them a skill to live by. For blind farmers increased training and resettlement grants are being given. New emphasis is being placed on employment for blind townspeople, for blind workshop and factory workers this means diversifying trades and improving marketing skills.

The Self Help Endowment (SHE) Fund, set up to meet the desperate need of blind women and girls, in many countries, for family help and economic independence, now finances more than 50 projects.

Working on priority projects amongst some of the poorest communities in the world, the Society has already achieved a significant reduction in blindness throughout the Commonwealth and for the past 8 years has had the privilege of providing a central administration for IAPB.

Further information from: Royal Commonwealth Society for the Blind, Commonwealth House, Haywards Heath, West Sussex RH16 3AZ, UK.

Seva Foundation

The Seva Foundation is an international public health organization incorporated in 1978 and based in Chelsea, Michigan, USA. Seva's primary activities include the support of programmes to eliminate avoidable blindness through prevention of new cases and treatment of existing cases. Most of Seva's efforts have been directed toward working with blindness activities in Nepal and India.

In Nepal, Seva helped conduct a survey of blindness and blinding eye diseases as the basis for the WHO/Government of Nepal Blindness Programme. Seva continues to support this programme which includes the establishment of mobile eye care units, surgical treatment for cataract and trichiasis/entropion, and treatment for trachoma. An important component is the training of Nepalese ophthalmologists and ophthalmic assistants, as well as health education for primary eye care. With a population of under 15 million, Nepal has nearly as many blind persons as the entire USA. As the population ages, the numbers of people blind from cataract is likely to double in the next 20 years and as many as 300 000 sight-restoring operations may be needed.

In India, Seva provides support to the Aravind Eye Hospital in Madurai, South India. Founded in 1976 as a 20-bed hospital by Dr G. Venkataswamy, Aravind has grown rapidly and now houses up to 500 patients, about 75 per cent of whom are treated free of cost. To date over 22 000 people have benefited from free cataract surgery, and over 200 000 have been examined and treated for various eye ailments. Aravind also screens children for malnutrition and vitamin-A deficiency and, where necessary, treats them to prevent blindness. Seva has helped in making Aravind's excellent services more widely available through consultants, training in epidemiology and hospital administration, health education studies, and small 'seed' grants.

Seva is committed to the alleviation of suffering through the appropriate use of science and technology, seeking to provide technical and financial support to projects which aim to control the causes of curable and preventable blindness such as cataract, trachoma, and vitamin-A-deficiency blindness.

Seva sees its role as a catalyst, providing initial 'seed' grants to help get programmes underway or to help them to extend in new directions, and then continuing its support by helping to provide the kinds of services not otherwise available. Seva is not a large scale fund-raising organization, it relies heavily on volunteers and on in-kind donations to fill the needs in the programmes they support.

Further information from: SEVA, 108 Spring Lake Drive, Chelsea, MI 48118, USA.

Appendix I

INTERNATIONAL AGENCY FOR THE PREVENTION OF BLINDNES

Headquarters: National Eye Institute, Building 31, Room 6A03, Bethesda, Maryland 20205, USA.

Officers of the Agency

The following officers were elected at the Second General Assembly in October 1982:

President:	Dr Carl Kupfer
Honorary President:	Sir John Wilson
Vice Presidents:	President of the International Federation of Ophthalmological Societies
	President of the World Council for the Welfare of the Blind
	Director-General of the World Health Organization (or nominee)
	Professor Barrie R. Jones
Treasurer:	Dr W. S. Hunter
Registrar/Secretary:	Dr V. Clemmesen

Regional Chairmen

The following Regional Chairmen were elected at the Second General Assembly in October 1982:

Africa	Professor C. O. Quarcoopome, Head of Ophthalmology Department, University of Ghana Medical School, PO Box 4236, Accra, Ghana.
Eastern Europe	Colonel Boris Zimin, President of the World Council for the Welfare of the Blind, Novaja Plochad 14, Moscow, USSR.
Latin America	Dr F. C. Contreras, Director, Centro Oftalmologico, 'Luciano Barrere' Hospital Santo Toribio de Mogrovejo, Ancash 1271, Lima, Peru.
Middle East	Sheikh Abdullah Al-Ghanim, Chairman, The Regional Bureau of the Middle East Committee for the Welfare of the Blind, PO Box 3465, Riyadh, Saudi Arabia.
North America	Mrs V. Boyce, c/o National Society to Prevent Blindness, 79 Madison Avenue, New York, NY 10016-7896, USA.
South East Asia	Dr A. Lim, 0609, Mt Elizabeth Medical Centre, Mt Elizabeth, Singapore 0922.

Southern Asia   Dr R. Pararajasegaram,
Medical Officer Prevention of Blindness for
Regional Director WHO,
World Health Organization,
Regional Office for South-East Asia,
World Health House, New Delhi,
1.10.002, India.

Western Europe   Professor Jules Francois,
15 Place de Smet de Naeyer, B-9000,
Ghent, Belgium.

Western Pacific Professor A. Nakajima,
Professor and Chairman,
Department of Ophthalmology,
Juntendo University Medical School,
3-1-3 Hongo Bunkyo-Ku, Tokyo, Japan.

Members of the Executive Board

Group A: Members appointed on the nomination of the International Council of Ophthalmology to represent organizations concerned with opthalmology and with the prevention of blindness.

Dr Carl Kupfer, National Eye Institute, Building 31, Room 6A03, Bethesda, Maryland 20205, USA.

Professor Barrie R. Jones, International Centre for Eye Health, Institute of Ophthalmology, University of London, 27/29 Cayton Street, London EC1V 2PD, UK.
(Alternate: Dr Bjorn Thylefors, Prevention of Blindness Programme, World Health Organization, 1211 Geneva 27, Switzerland.)

Professor Jules Francois, 15 Place de Smet de Naeyer, B-9000, Ghent, Belgium.

Dr Viggo Clemmesen, Chr. Winthers Vej 28, 4700 Naestved, Denmark.
(Alternate: Dr Branko Nizetic, Regional Office for Europe, World Health Organization, 8 Scherfigs-Vej, 2100 Copenhagen Ø, Denmark.)

Professor Akira Nakajima, Department of Ophthalmology, Juntendo University School of Medicine, 3-1-3 Hongo, Bunkyo-Ku, Tokyo, Japan.
(Alternate: Professor Hsiao-Lou Chang, Director Beijing Institute of Ophthalmology, Tong Ren Hospital, Beijing, People's Republic of China.)

Group B: Members appointed on the nomination of the World Council for the Welfare of the Blind and the International Federation of the Blind to represent organizations of and for the blind:

Colonel Boris Zimin, President, World Council for the Welfare of the Blind, Novaja Plochad 14, Moscow, USSR.
(Alternate: Mr John C. Colligan, 3 Jonathans, Dene Road, Northwood, Middlesex HA6 2AD, UK.)

Senora Dorina de Gouvea Nowill, Fundacao para o Livro do Cego No Brasil, Caixa Postal no. 20.384, Rua Dr. Diogo de Faria 558, 04037 Sao Paulo, Brazil.
(Alternate: Mr E. T. Boulter, Royal National Institute for the Blind, 224 Great Portland Street, London, W1N 6AA, UK.)

Sheikh Abdullah M. Al-Ghanim, The Regional Bureau of the Middle East Committee for the Welfare of the Blind, PO Box 3465, Riyadh, Saudi Arabia.

Dr F. Sonntag, President Bund der Kriegsblinden Deutschlands e.V., Schumannstrasse 35, 5300 Bonn, Federal Republic of Germany.
(Alternate: Mr Suresh Ahuja, Executive Officer, National Association for the Blind, 51 Mahatma Gandhi Road, Bombay 400 023, India.)

The nominee and the alternate of the IFB to be appointed.

Group C: Members elected to represent national delegations:

Dr R. Pararajasegaram, World Health Organization, Regional Office for South East Asia, World Health House, New Delhi 1.10.002, India.
(Alternate: Professor R. Siva Reddy, Lalitha Nilayam, 3-5-886 Himayat Nagar, Hyderabad, 500 029, India.)

Professor C. O. Quarcoopome, University of Ghana Medical School, Unit of Ophthalmology, PO Box 4236, Accra, Ghana.
(Alternate: Dr Chirambo, Ministry of Health, PO Box 30377, Lilongwe 3, Malawi.)

Dr Hadi El-Sheikh, Associate Professor of Ophthalmology, Khartoum Eye Hospital, Faculty of Medicine, PO Box 1012, Khartoum, Sudan.
(Alternate: Dr Sabri Kamel, 44 Opera Square, Cairo, Egypt.)

Dr Francisco Contreras, Hospital Santo Toribio de Mogrovejo, Servicio de Oftalmologia, Ancash 1271, Lima, Peru.
(Alternate: Senora Molina de Stahl, Comite Nacional Pro-Ciegos Y Sordomudos, 4a Avenida 2-28, Zona 1, Guatemala, Central America.)

Dr Arthur Lim, 0609, Mt. Elizabeth Medical Centre, Mt. Elizabeth, Singapore 0922.

Dr A. Dubois-Poulsen, 8 Avenue Daniel Le Sueur, Paris, 7, France.

Group D: Members elected to represent scientific disciplines other than ophthalmology:

Mr L. Teply, UNICEF, United Nations, New York 10017, USA.
(Alternate: Dr A. Sommer, International Centre for Epidemiologic and Preventive Ophthalmology, The Wilmer Institute, Baltimore, Maryland 21205, USA.)

Dr C. Dawson, Francis I. Proctor Foundation for Research in Ophthalmology, University of California, Third and Parnassus, San Francisco, California 94122, USA.
(Alternate: Dr F. Hollows, Department of Ophthalmology, Prince of Wales Hospital, Randwick, New South Wales—2031, Australia.)

Dr L. Brilliant, University of Michigan, Department of Epidemiology, 109 Observatory Street, Ann Arbor, Michigan 48109, USA.
(Alternate: Dr N. Grasset, Les Champs Fleuris, Veigy-Foncenex, Douvaine 74 140, France.)

Dr Venkataswamy, Aravind Eye Hospital, 1 Housing Board Colony, Sathamangalam, Madurai 625 020, India.
(Alternate: Dr Harry King Jnr., The International Eye Foundation, 7801 Norfolk Avenue, Bethesda, Maryland, 20014, USA.)

Group E: Members representing the following international non-governmental organizations:

Asian Foundation for the Prevention of Blindness
Christoffel Blindenmission
Helen Keller International
International Organization Against Trachoma
Royal Commonwealth Society for the Blind

(Provision has been made for the election of up to five more organizations, on the recommendation of the organizations presently elected.)

Group F: Members 'at large' elected in recognition of the individual contributions which they can make to the work of the Agency:

Dr W. J. Holmes, 3885 Round Top Drive, Honolulu, Hawaii 96822, USA.
(Alternate: Dr K. Kaiser-Kupfer, National Eye Institute, Building 31, Bethesda, Maryland 20205, USA.)

Mrs V. Boyce, National Society to Prevent Blindness, 79 Madison Avenue, New York, NY 10016-7896, USA.
(Alternate: Mr R. Mercer, Canadian National Institute for the Blind, 1929 Bay View Avenue, Toronto, Ontario, Canada M4G 3E8.)

Dr W. S. Hunter, 600 Sherbourne Street, Suite 812, Toronto, Ontario M4X 1W4, Canada.

Professor Madan Mohan, Dr Rajendra Prasad Centre for Ophthalmic Sciences, Ansari Nagar, New Delhi—110016, India.

Dr F. Billson, Department of Clinical Ophthalmology, Sydney Eye Hospital, Sir John Young Crescent, Woolloomooloo 2011, Australia.

Dr A. E. Maumenee, The Wilmer Institute, Johns Hopkins Hospital, Baltimore, Maryland, 21205, USA.
(Alternate: Lady Wilson, Royal Commonwealth Society for the Blind, Commonwealth House, Haywards Heath, West Sussex RH16 3AZ, UK.)

Appendix II

LIST OF PARTICIPANTS

Dr M. M. Abdou *Nigeria*
Dr E. O. Akinsete *Nigeria*
Sheikh Abdullah Al-Ghanim *Saudi Arabia*
Professor Aliou Bah *Mali*
Mr S. A-Almajid *Saudi Arabia*
Professor M. N. Amin *Bangladesh*
Dr Arenas Archila *Colombia*
Dr A. M. Awan *Kenya*
Dr Ibrahim Ayesh *Jordan*
Ms M. B. Ayldon *USA*

Dr Bambang *Indonesia*
Dr Beltranena *Guatemala*
Dr Benjelloun *Morocco*
Mr Bruce Benson *USA*
Professor Frank Billson *Australia*
Dr Bitran *Chile*
Dr J. van Bochove *Netherlands Antilles*
Dr J. Boisson *France*
Dr Bon Sol Koo *Korea*
Dr Breinin *USA*
Mrs Virginia Boyce *USA*
Miss Madli Brekke *USA*
Dr L. Brilliant *USA*
Dr Alfred Buck *USA*
Ms Kathe Burkhard *USA*

Dr J. Cadet *Haiti*
M Cambournac *France*
Mr L. Campbell *USA*
Dra de Carbonell *Venezuela*
Mr E. Timothy Carroll *USA*
Dr Eugene Chan *China*
Dr Girish Chandra *USA*
Dr G. Chester *Australia*
Mr David Chesterman *UK*
Dr M. C. Chirambo *Malawi*
Dr Monsur Ahmed Choudhuri *Bangladesh*
Dr Viggo Clemmesen *Denmark*
Dr David Cogan *USA*
Miss A. M. S. Connell *West Indies*
Dr Francisco Contreras *Peru*
Dr Copper *Netherlands*
Mr John Costello *USA*

Ms Ann Darnbrough *UK*
Dr Chandler R. Dawson *USA*
Dr Monteiro De Barros *Brazil*
Professor A. Dubois-Pulsen *France*

Dr El Gorafi *Yemen Arab Republic*
Dr Nicola Evtimov *Bulgaria*

Dr Mrs H. B. Faal *The Gambia*
Dr Fang Qian-Xun *China*
Professor Jules Francois *Belgium*
Mr Curtis Freeman *USA*

Dr Sudirojo Gambiro *Indonesia*
Mr E. Glaeser *USA*
Dr P. Graham *Australia*
Dr Griggs *USA*
Mr Richard Grove *USA*
Dr J. C. Gwasaze *Uganda*
Mr J. Gwayambadde *Uganda*

Mr P. Haegermalm *Sweden*
Dr E. Hansen *Norway*
Ms Dotty Harrell *USA*
Mr Sobhy Hassan *Egypt*
Dr Ralph Helmsen *USA*
Miss S. J. Hennighausen *Canada*
Dr Jens Hetland *Norway*
Dr Fred Hollows *Australia*
Dr Martin Holm *Sweden*
Dr W. J. Holmes *Hawaii*
Dr Rabiul Hussain *Bangladesh*
Miss Hutasoit *Indonesia*
Dr Hu Zheng *China*

Dr Herbert Insel *USA*
Dr Michael Irwin *USA*

Dr Jonathan Javitt *USA*
Dr A. T. Jenkyns *Canada*
Professor Barrie R. Jones *UK*

Dr Kaakinen *Finland*
Dr Sabri Kamel *Egypt*
Ms Margery Kenealy *USA*
Dr Kinabo *Tanzania*
Dr John Harry King Jr *USA*
Mr Lawrence M. King Jr *USA*
Dr T. J. Kirmani *Pakistan*
Dr V. Klauss *Kenya*
Dr Sidi Konare *Mali*
Monsieur Ismalia Konate *Mali*
Dr K. Kontturi *Finland*
Dr. A. Korra *Egypt*
Dr Kuo Pin-Kuan *China*
Dr Carl Kupfer *USA*
Dr Muriel Kaiser Kupfer *USA*
Dr Marvin Kwitko *Canada*

Dr Leo Landhuis *USA*
Dr Arthur S. M. Lim *Singapore*
Dr Erik Linner *Sweden*

Professor R. Mabrouk *Tunisia*
Mrs Lydia Mcguire *USA*
Mr E. McManus *USA*
Dr MacRery *USA*
Professor Mario Maione *Italy*
Dr Multafu Mangga *Nigeria*
Dr Yan Mangiwa *Indonesia*
Dr C. V. S. Mani *India*
Dr Winifred Mao *China*
Dr M. A. Matin *Bangladesh*
Dr Robert Meaders *USA*
Dr Vijay Mehra *India*
Miss K. Middleton *Haiti*
Dr C. Midy *Haiti*
Dr Roy Milton *USA*
Professor Madan Mohan *India*
Dr Reynold Monsanto *Haiti*
Dra Margarita Morales *Chile*
Mr Julian Morris *USA*
Dr Diaa Mosly *Saudi Arabia*
Dr M. P. Mphalele *South Africa*
Dr Raine Mustonen *Finland*

Dr Cameron Nabeel *Jordan*
Professor Akira Nakajima *Japan*
Dr Negrel *France*
Dr Ne Yong Shin *South Korea*
Dr David Nicolle *Canada*

Dr Oyin Olurin *Nigeria*
Dr Olabopo Osuntokun *Nigeria*
Dr Victor Segun Oyeleye *Nigeria*

Professor Pahwa *India*
Dr R. Pararajasegaram *India*
Dr Paul *India*
Dr Susan Pettiss *USA*
Dr B. Philipson *Sweden*
Dr Pielasch *East Germany*
Dr Pillay *Mauritius*
Dr and Mrs George Porter *USA*
Mrs R. Powell *Guatemala*
Mr Pitts Crick *UK*

Professor C. P. Quarcoopome *Ghana*

Dr Rafii *Morocco*
Padmabhusan Professor Dr P. Siva
  Reddy *India*
Mrs Lila Rosenblum *USA*
Mr W. P. Rowland *South Africa*

Professor I. S. Roy *India*

Ms Salqvist *Sweden*
Dr Fouad Sayegh *Jordan*
Mr Larry T. Schwab *USA*
Ms Victoria Sheffield *USA*
Dr Shukla *Zambia*
Mr Abu Siddique *Bangladesh*
Mr Arnold Simonse *USA*
Dr Eugene So *USA*
Dr Alfred Sommer *USA*
Mrs E. Molina de Stahl *Guatemala*
Mr W. Stein *West Germany*
Dr A. A. Stulting *South Africa*
Dr K. L. Stumpf *Hong Kong*
Dr J. W. Swartwood *USA*

Dr I. Tarwotjo *Indonesia*
Dr Hugh Taylor *USA*
Dr Joseph Taylor *Tanzania*
Professor Main Tell *Jordan*
Dr Johanna Ten Doesschate *Netherlands*
Dr L. Teply *USA*
Dr Bjorn Thylefors *Switzerland*
Mr Robert Tilden *USA*
Mr Teferra Tizazu *USA*
Dr Asbjorn M. Tonjum *Norway*
Sr Evelyn Tremblay *Haiti*
Ms Gloria Tujab *Guatemala*

Dr Upadhyay *Nepal*
Dr W. Utomo *Indonesia*

Mr S. T. van der Walt *South Africa*
Dr Don P. Vandyke *USA*
Dr G. Venkataswamy *India*
Padhma Sri Dr R. Vyas *India*

Dr E. Wagner *West Germany*
Mrs A. Warwick *UK*
Mr Aubrey Webson *West Indies*
Dr Randolph Whitfield *USA*
Mrs B. Wick *East Germany*
Mr J. W. Wilson *Australia*
Sir John Wilson *UK*
Lady Wilson *UK*
Dr Frank Winter *USA*

Professor Dr Yin Su Yun *China*

Dr Pedro Zurita *Spain*

Index

Accra 20
Africa 4, 6, 10, 15, 18, 19, 20, 21
AFRO (African Regional Office of the WHO) 20
Al-Ghanim, Sheik Abdullah, M. 32
All Russia Association of the Blind 26
Alma Ata 17
Al Nur Institute 35
American Pharmaceutical Association 38
Amman 36
Andheri Hilfe 45
Arab Gulf Programme 16
Arafat 35
Aravind Eye Hospital 48, 80, 100
Asia 5, 10, 15
Aswan Foundation for the Prevention of Blindness 41, 42, 43, 101
Association of Surgeons of East Africa 74
Australia 40, 45, 50, 51, 53, 112
Awan, Dr A. M. 70

Baghdad 14
Baltimore 16, 41
Bamako 20
Bangladesh 6, 40, 43, 44, 45, 50, 53, 98, 99
Bangkok 42
Barbados 29
Bhutan 43, 46, 98
Billson, Professor 50
Blantyre 68, 69
Botswana 20, 21
Boyce, Virginia 36
Brazil 10, 29
Briscoe, Gordon 51
Bulgaria 25, 26
Burma 44, 46, 98, 99
Burroughs Wellcome Fund 39

Canada 22, 30, 31, 36, 37, 40, 48, 79, 103
Caribbean 29
cataract vii, 8, 9, 10, 13, 15, 19, 21, 22, 23, 24, 27, 33, 35, 36, 37, 40, 41, 42, 44, 48, 52, 53, 54, 58, 62, 71, 72, 81, 85, 86, 92
Center for Disease Control, Atlanta, USA 79
Chen Yao-Zhen 92
Chile 29
China, People's Republic of 10, 52, 53, 78, 92
Chirambo, M. C. 67

Chittagong 45, 50
cholera 57
Christoffel Blindenmission 16, 48, 53, 59, 79
Clemmesen, Dr Viggo 49
Collaborating Centres for the Prevention of Blindness (WHO) 16, 29, 30, 100, 110
Colombia 30
Contreras, Dr Francisco 13, 29, 82
Cornell University 97
Costa Rica 30
Costello, J. H. 95
Coster, Professor 53
Cuellar, Perez de 1
Czechoslovakia 27

Dawson, Dr C. 13, 34
Dhaka 45
diabetes 19, 27, 37, 49, 51
Dr Rajendra Prasad Centre for Ophthalmic Sciences 47
Dr Rodolfo Robles Hospital 30

East Africa 6
Eastern Europe 15, 24
Egypt 32, 34, 35
Ethiopia 20
Europe 112

Fiji 51, 52, 53
Flinders University 53
Flying Doctor Service 69
foresight 50, 53
France 79
Francis, I. Proctor Foundation 34

Gambia 20, 21, 22
Garoka 53
Geneva 101
German Democratic Republic 27
Ghana 10, 20, 21
glaucoma vii, 10, 11, 13, 15, 19, 21, 22, 24-9, 33, 35-8, 42, 44, 46, 49, 51-4, 62, 92
Grasset, Dr Nicole 78
Greece 49
Greenland 49
Guan Zheng-she 92
Guatemala 6, 30, 53, 89, 92
Guinea-Bissau 20
Gurkha soldiers 79

Haiti 30

Index

Harare 24
Helen Keller International 16, 30, 31, 40, 42, 48, 49, 53, 84, 88, 89, 96, 97
Hollows, Professor Fred 51, 74
Hong Kong 41, 52, 112
Hungary 25, 27
Hyderabad 87

impact 17
India 4, 6, 9, 15, 44, 45, 46, 47, 48, 55, 58, 59, 78, 80, 81, 82, 98, 99, 100
Indonesia 6, 41, 86, 87, 88, 89
International Agency for the Prevention of Blindness (IAPB) vii, 1-5, 10, 14, 15, 16, 18, 37, 41, 45, 48, 50, 55, 59, 93, 94, 95, 103, 106, 107, 109, 111-14
International Eye Foundation 16, 20, 21, 40, 69
International Federation of the Blind 110
International Federation of Ophthalmic Societies 16
International Organization Against Trachoma 14, 16
International Vitamin A Consultative Group 21
International Year of the Child 17, 34
International Year of Disabled Persons 1, 2, 17, 34

Jakarta 89
Japan 16, 52, 53, 79, 112
Japan Shipbuilding Industry Foundation 79, 101
Japanese Glaucoma Research Association 38
Java 87
Jenkyns, A. T. 102
Jordan 32, 35, 36

Karachi 36
Kathmandu 78-80
Kenya 7, 18, 20, 21, 22, 69, 70, 71, 73, 74
keratomalacia 5, 54
Klauss, Dr Volker 70, 74
Korimbo, Dr Peter 53
Kupfer, Dr Carl vii, 4, 13, 71, 72, 114

Latin America 15, 29
Lesotho 20, 21, 22
Liberia 20, 22
Lilongwe 20, 68, 69
Lim, Dr A. S. M. 40, 41, 50, 111
Lima 83
Linner, Dr 13
Lions Clubs 13, 77, 86, 100
London 16, 41

Madurai 48, 80
Mahidol University 42
malaria 57
Malawi 20, 22, 23, 67, 68, 69
Malaysia 42
Maldives 44, 48, 98, 99, 100
Mali 20
Manila 53
Mao Wen-shu 92
Meaders, R. H. 60
Mexico 31
Middle East 4, 15, 32, 33
Mohan, Madan 55
Morocco 32
Morse, Bradford 1
Mudaliar Committee 57
Muller, Dr Robert 1, 114
Muscat 33

Nairobi 21
Nakajima, Professor 13, 50
National Eye Institute, USA 114
Nepal 44, 48, 78, 79, 80, 98, 99, 100
Netherlands 16
New Delhi 43
Nigeria 20, 21
North America 36, 37, 40, 112
Norway 16
Nowill, Dorina de Gouvêa 108
Nutritional blindness 19, 58; see also xerophthalmia

ocular trauma 12, 13, 15, 19, 21, 22, 23, 24, 27, 36, 53, 62
Oman 33
Ommen, Professor 86
onchocerciasis 7, 8, 13, 14, 15, 19, 23, 30, 32, 33, 53
Onchocerciasis, Control Programme 7, 8, 20, 21
Operation Eyesight Universal 16, 22, 30, 31, 40, 46, 48, 79, 84, 102
Operation YELEEN 23
Organization of American States 110
Organizacion Panamericana de la Salud see PAHO

Pakistan 35, 82
Pan American Health Organization (PAHO) 29, 96
Papua New Guinea 51, 52, 53
Pararajasegaram, Dr R. 43, 78, 97
Peru 31, 82, 97
Pettiss, Dr Susan 89
Philippines 51, 53
Pirie, Dr 111
Pokhrel, Dr R. P. 78
Port-au-Prince 30
Port Moresby University 53

Index 137

Programme Advisory Groups on the Prevention of Blindness (WHO) 3, 13, 16
Project Orbis 41

Quarcoopome, Professor 13, 18

Rajendra Prasad Centre for Ophthalmic Sciences 100
Rangoon 46
Red Cross 13, 100, 103
Regional Ophthalmic Academy 16
Riyadh 34
Rotary Clubs 13, 86, 100
Royal Australian College of Ophthalmologists 51
Royal Commonwealth Society for the Blind 9, 16, 21, 36, 43, 45, 46, 47, 48, 49, 53, 59, 79, 85, 86, 101
Rumania 25, 28

Sahelian belt 19
San Fransisco 16, 34
Sarahsawa Shipbuilding Foundation 53
Sarojini Devi Eye Hospital 100
Saudi Arabia 32, 33, 34
Senegal 20
Seva Foundation 16, 40, 78
sickle cell disease 19
Sierra Leone 20, 21, 22
Singapore 40, 41, 42, 45, 111
smallpox 25, 57
Solomon Islands 52, 54
Sommer, Dr 13, 89
South-East Asia 4, 10, 40, 41, 43, 50, 111
South-East Asian Fluorescein Angiography Club 40
South Korea 54
Southern Asia 15, 43, 44, 97, 100
Soviet Union see USSR
Sri Lanka 43, 45, 48, 97, 98, 99, 100
Steinkuller, Dr Paul 71
Stumpf, Karl 103
Sudan 19, 20, 32
Swaziland 20, 23
Swiss Red Cross 79
Syria 32

Tanzania 97
Tarwotjo, I. 86, 89
Thailand 42, 51
Thuku, Dr J. J. 70
Tilden, Robert 86
Togo 20, 23
trachoma, 4, 5, 13, 14, 15, 17, 19, 21-5, 27, 30, 32, 33, 35, 36, 44, 46, 47, 49, 51, 54, 57, 58, 63, 75, 92
tuberculosis 57
Tujab 89

UNESCO 1, 3, 110
UNICEF 17, 45, 101, 110, 111
United Kingdom 45
United Nations 1, 2, 3, 16, 98, 101, 112
United Nations Development Programme (UNDP) 17, 46, 101
United States Agency for International Development (USAID) 21, 89, 96
United States of America (USA) vii, 10, 12, 16, 36, 37, 38, 40, 41, 103, 114
University of Alexandria 34
University of California 34
University of Jordan 35
USSR 24-7, 54
uveitis 19, 23

veneral diseases 25, 27
Venezuela 31
Vietnam 54
Vision 41, 111, 113
Volta River Basin 7, 8, 20
Vyas, Rajendra T. 85

West Germany 45
West Indies 113
Western Europe 49
Western Pacific 15, 50
WHO (World Health Organization) vii, 1, 2, 3, 13, 14, 15, 16, 17, 20, 22, 32, 35, 36, 40, 42, 43, 46, 48, 49, 52, 53, 78, 84, 89, 92, 96, 100, 101, 102, 110, 111, 112, 115
WHO Collaborating Centres for the Prevention of Blindness see Collaborating Centres
WHO Expanded Programme on Immunization 22
WHO (World Health Organization) Regional Committee for Africa 20, 21
Whitfield, R. 69
Wilson, Lady 110
Wilson, Sir John 14, 55, 114
World blindness and its prevention 111
World Congress of Ophthalmology 16
World Council for the Welfare of the Blind 16, 110
World Health Organization, see WHO

xerophthalmia 5, 6, 13, 15, 17, 30, 40, 41, 44, 53, 58, 86, 87, 88, 89
Xerophthalmia Bulletin 111

Yemen Arab Republic 32, 36
Yugoslavia 28

Zambia 20, 24
Zimbabwe 20, 24
Zimin, Colonel Boris 24

DATE DUE

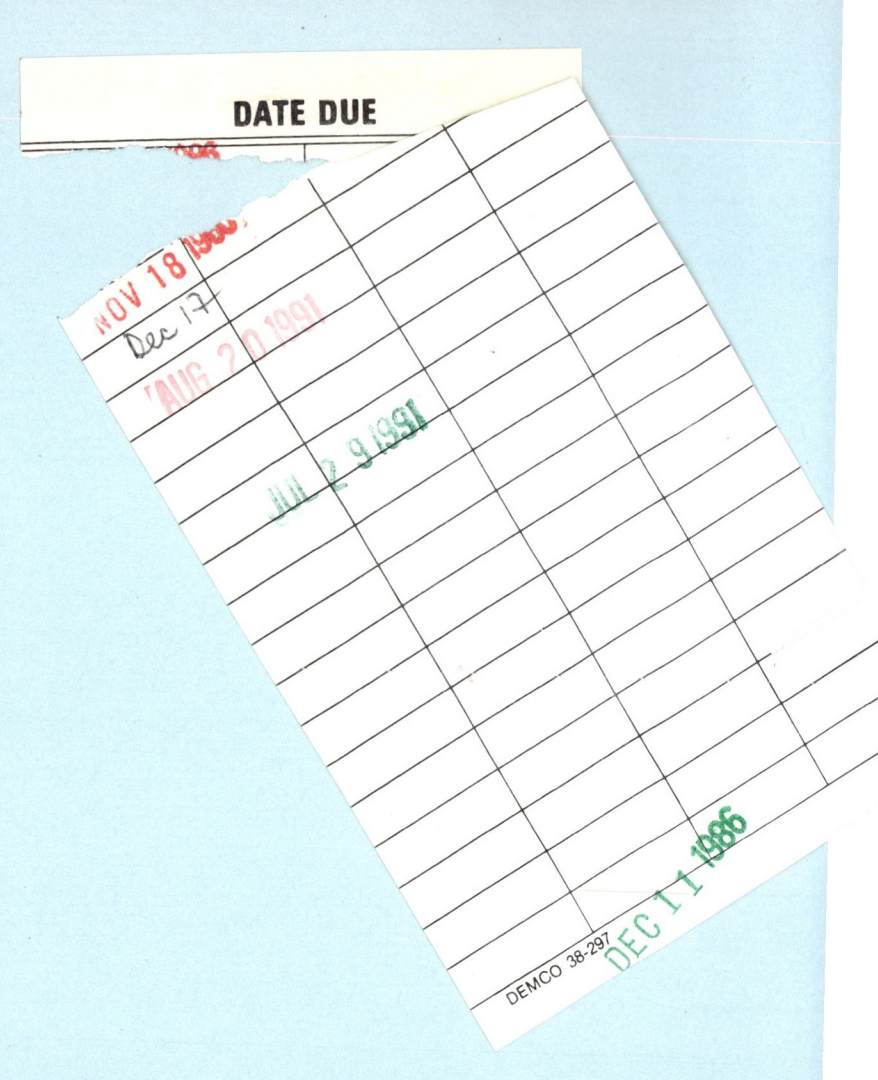

NOV 18
Dec 17
AUG 20 1991
JUL 2 9 1991
DEC 11 1986

DEMCO 38-297

3 1211 00806695 9